Bioencapsulation of Living Cells for Diverse Medical Applications

Editors

Eva Maria Brandtner

Vorarlberg Institute for Vascular Investigation and Treatment (VIVIT)
Austria

&

John Austin Dangerfield

SG Austria/Austrianova Singapore
Singapore

CONTENTS

FOREWORD

It is almost 60 years since the first successful organ transplantation, which took place in 1954, revolutionised medicine. Since then, the idea of implanting living cells, tissues and organs into the body has been pursued as a strategy for the treatment of a variety of diseases. Microencapsulation of cells and their implantation into the body can be viewed as an extension or specialised form of organ transplantation in that it allows cells to take over a missing or defective function in the body. However, unlike organ transplantation, microencapsulation has the advantage that immunosuppression is not needed due to the immunoprotective effects of the encapsulation material, which also acts as a safety device. Microencapsulation of cells can be achieved using a number of different polymers, most notably alginate, cellulose sulphate and agarose, all of which are included in the various chapters that comprise this eBook. Excitingly, microencapsulated cells are already more than living up to their potential in that they have been shown to be safe and efficacious in numerous clinical trials, and this is regardless of the encapsulation material used. Our major contribution to this field was the first clinical trial that employed cellulose sulphate encapsulated cells for the treatment of pancreatic cancer.

The editors of this timely eBook and my dear colleagues and friends, Dr. Eva Maria Brandtner and Dr. John Dangerfield, have brought together contributions from some of the leading research in the field of cell encapsulation with the aim of providing an overview of the status of the latest exciting developments. The use of implanted, microencapsulated cells has long been proposed as a means to treat a variety of diseases but has historically mainly focussed on diabetes which is still a major focus for many academic groups and companies (as is reviewed in this eBook in the chapters by Tuch and Vaithilingam as well as that by Bilodeau and Halle). However, encapsulated cells are being used to treat a wide variety of diseases and now are even being used to improve on stem cell therapies which have generally been proposed as a cell based, cure all. Here the capsule material functions as both a safety device, as well as a means to localise cells to the site where they are needed. Encapsulation may help cells survive longer as well as prevent immune rejection and/or Graft *vs.* Host Disease, the most common adverse event seen in stem cell clinical trials. As evidenced by the chapters in this exciting new eBook, great progress has been made in improving the survival of encapsulated cells as well as moving these novel therapies into the clinic.

As well as use in cancer therapy to improve on existing chemotherapies by reducing the dose and thus side effects while increasing efficacy (see chapters by Dangerfield and colleagues and also by Sakai and co-workers), encapsulated cells can be used to produce antibodies. These can be tumoricidal antibodies or virus neutralising activities. The advantages of using encapsulated cells rather than more conventional injections as a delivery means include the long term stable and steady state levels that result from production of antibodies by implanted encapsulated cells.

CNS diseases such as epilepsy, neurodegenerative disorders like Parkinson's disease, Alzheimer, Amyotrophic lateral sclerosis, Huntington's disease but also pathologies caused by trauma and/or ischemic processes and brain tumors are ideal candidates for treatment using encapsulated cells producing neuron nurturing factors and this is the focus of the chapter by López-Méndez and colleagues.

Cell types that have been encapsulated for therapeutic purposes include islet cells, stem cells and "platform" cell lines such as HEK293 and CHO cells. Stem cells are of particular interest. Two of the chapters discuss the use of encapsulated stem cells. Tuch and Vaithilingam discuss the use of pancreatic progenitors from pluripotent human embryonic stem cells as a much more reliable and larger source of surrogate cells for encapsulation and transplantation than human or porcine islets which are in limited supply and more likely to be contaminated with adventitious agents.

Inducible expression and expression control may or may not be required, depending on the disease and whether there are dosing issues. Islet cells have the intrinsic ability to sense glucose levels and to respond by producing insulin when glucose levels are high or not when levels are low. Genetic engineering of cells can allow control of expression of biotherapeutic products from encapsulated cells. Ortner, Kaspar and Czerny review some of the methods used to achieve inducible or controllable gene expression, including a novel system that they have pioneered using heat as the inducer of expression.

While I am sure this will not be the last word (or eBook) on this exciting and fast moving field of cell microencapsulation, I think this eBook will be much more than a useful resource for all researchers, clinicians and those interested in the future of biomedicine. Well done Lilli, John and the various colleagues and friends who have contributed to this excellent eBook.

Brian Salmons

SG Austria/Austrianova Singapore
Singapore

PREFACE

The encapsulation of cells into a biocompatible shell has three main purposes: 1) Protection of the cells from the immunity of the living system where they are applied 2) Physical localisation of the cells, and hence the biomolecule they produce, at the therapeutic target site (in contrast to single cells which would in most cases migrate or move away at some point) and 3) The opportunity to remove the cells after treatment is completed if required.

The concept of encapsulation to allow implantation of foreign cells into a patient is not new, but is something that has still not been successfully developed to the point at which a licensed medical product exists on the market. In times when allogeneic cell therapy is considered to be potentially big business and encapsulation allows an easy way to make a "one-for-all" product, this is surprising. This is most likely due to the complex challenges of generating a GMP (Good Manufacturing Practice) grade of off-the-shelf living cell product in addition to the challenges of combining this with an encapsulation device. Several research laboratories and small companies are however currently working to achieve this with some varying levels of success. An Australian based company named Living Cell Technologies has achieved small scale GMP production and is undertaking clinical trials for the treatment of diabetes and has encouraging pre-clinical work for a number of other neurodegenerative applications. The US based company Novocell also has a focus on stem cell encapsulation for diabetes treatment and a clinical trial has been undertaken. The now Singapore based company, SG Austria (Austrianova Singapore), could show safety and efficacy of encapsulated cells producing a prodrug converting enzyme in a clinical phase I/II trial for pancreatic cancer (Lohr *et al.*, 2001). Subsequently, orphan drug status was granted and a large-scale GMP facility with production license was established, showing for the first time that it could be done (Salmons *et al.*, 2007). More recently in 2012, they presented similar positive results for a second phase II trial in the same indication.

Proof of principle has been shown for several different encapsulation techniques and materials (and combinations thereof). Predominantly, biocompatible and nontoxic polymers such as sodium cellulose sulphate, alginate, agarose or polyethylene glycol are used. The speed and sterility of the process and the quality and purity of the encapsulation agents are critical for success and reproducibility of the procedure and further viability of the cells, *i.e.,* that they continue to produce and/or secrete their therapeutically relevant biomolecules and remain bio-inert when implanted into animals or patients.

A huge variety of cells with proven or potential therapeutic activity exist in research laboratories and companies alike and because many of these cells cannot be brought into the patient directly such groups are networking hard with encapsulation specialists. A prominent example is the use of pig islet cells, or other forms of insulin producing cells, for the treatment of diabetes. In immune deficient animal models such cells can react to blood sugar levels and produce insulin on demand, and encapsulation offers the perfect way to bring such cells into a patient.

This eBook describes the details and pros and cons of the currently most used and most promising types of encapsulation methods and materials as well as the currently most focused-on cells, biomolecules and disease areas. Authored by leading scientists and company executives, it gives relevant examples, reviews published data and describes the projects closest to commercialisation. Several chapters also include easy-to-follow lab protocols making it a useful laboratory handbook for researchers and students alike.

Eva Maria Brandtner

Vorarlberg Institute for Vascular Investigation and Treatment (VIVIT)
Austria

&

John Austin Dangerfield

SG Austria/Austrianova Singapore
Singapore

List of Contributors

Abastado, Jean-Pierre. Singapore Immunology Network (SIgN), 8A Biomedical Grove, Immunos Building, Level 4, 138648, Singapore.

Arii, Shigeki. Department of Hepato-Biliary-Pancreatic Surgery, Graduate School of Medicine, Tokyo Medical and Dental University 1-5-45 Yushima, Bunkyo-ku, Tokyo 113-8519, Japan.

Bilodeau, Stéphanie. University of Montreal/Centre Research Hospital Maisonneuve-Rosemont Research Laboratory on Bio-artificial Therapies, 5415 boul. L'Assomption, Montreal (Quebec), H1T 2M4, Canada.

Brandtner, Eva Maria. Vorarlberg Institute for Vascular Investigation and Treatment (VIVIT), Molecular Biology Laboratory, Stadtstrasse 33, A-6850 Dornbirn, Austria.

Corteling, Randolph. ReNeuron Limited, 10 Nugent Road, Surrey Research Park, Guildford, GU2 7AF, Surrey, UK.

Czerny, Thomas. University of Applied Sciences, FH Campus Wien, Department for Applied Life Sciences, Helmut-Qualtinger-Gasse 2, A-1030 Vienna, Austria

Dangerfield, John Austin. SG Austria/Austrianova Singapore, 20 Biopolis Way, #05-518 Centros, 138668, Singapore.

Foster, Jayne. Former Diabetes Transplant Unit, Prince of Wales Hospital & University of New South Wales, Sydney, Australia.

Gunzburg, Walter. SG Austria/Austrianova Singapore, 20 Biopolis Way, #05-518 Centros, Singapore 138668 ; Institute of Virology in the Department of Pathobiology, University of Veterinary Medicine, A-1220 Vienna, Austria.

Hallé, Jean-Pierre. University of Montreal/Centre Research Hospital Maisonneuve-Rosemont/Laboratory Research on Bio-artificial Therapies, 5415 boul. L'Assomption, Montreal (Quebec), H1T 2M4, Canada.

Hernández, Rosa Martin. NanoBioCel Group, Laboratory of Pharmaceutics, University of the Basque Country, School of Pharmacy, Vitoria-Gasteiz, Spain.

Kaspar, Cornelius. Department for Pathobiology, Institute of Virology, University of Veterinary Medicine, Veterinärplatz 1, A-1210 Vienna, Austria.

Kawakami, Koei. Department of Chemical Engineering, Faculty of Engineering, Kyushu University, 744 Motooka, Nishi-ku, Fukuoka, 819-0395, Japan.

López-Méndez, Tania. NanoBioCel Group, Laboratory of Pharmaceutics, University of the Basque Country, School of Pharmacy, Vitoria-Gasteiz, Spain.

Murua, Ainhoa. NanoBioCel Group, Laboratory of Pharmaceutics, University of the Basque Country, School of Pharmacy, Vitoria-Gasteiz, Spain; Networking Biomedical Research Center on Bioengineering, Biomaterials and Nanomedicine, CIBER-BBN, Vitoria-Gasteiz, Spain.; Laboratory of Pharmaceutical Technology, School of Pharmacy, University of the Basque Country, Paseo de la Universidad street 7, 01006 Vitoria-Gasteiz, Spain.

Orive, Gorka Arroyo. NanoBioCel Group, Laboratory of Pharmaceutics, University of the Basque Country, School of Pharmacy, Vitoria-Gasteiz, Spain.

Ortner, Viktoria. University of Applied Sciences, FH Campus Wien, Department for Applied Life Sciences, Helmut-Qualtinger-Gasse 2, A-1030 Vienna, Austria.

Pedraz Muñoz, José Luis. NanoBioCel Group, Laboratory of Pharmaceutics, University of the Basque Country, School of Pharmacy, Vitoria-Gasteiz, Spain.

Salmons, Brian. SG Austria/Austrianova Singapore, 20 Biopolis Way, #05-518 Centros, 138668, Singapore.

Shinji, Sakai. Department of Materials Science and Engineering, Graduate School of Engineering Science, Osaka University, 1-3 Machikaneyama-cho, Toyonaka, Osaka 560-8531, Japan.

Sinden, John. ReNeuron Limited, 10 Nugent Road, Surrey Research Park, Guildford, GU2 7AF, Surrey, UK.

Tanaka, Shinji. Department of Hepato-Biliary-Pancreatic Surgery, Graduate School of Medicine, Tokyo Medical and Dental University 1-5-45 Yushima, Bunkyo-ku, Tokyo 113-8519, Japan.

Tuch, Bernard. Biomedical Materials & Devices, Materials, Science & Engineering, Commonwealth Scientific & Industrial Research Organization (CSIRO), Riverside, Life Science Centre, 11 Julius Avenue, North Ryde, NSW 2113, Australia; former Diabetes Transplant Unit, Prince of Wales Hospital & University of New South Wales, Sydney, Australia.

Vaithilingam, Vijayaganapathy. Biomedical Materials & Devices, Materials, Science & Engineering, Commonwealth Scientific & Industrial Research Organization (CSIRO), Riverside, Life Science Centre, 11 Julius Avenue, North Ryde, NSW 2113, Australia; former Diabetes Transplant Unit, Prince of Wales Hospital & University of New South Wales, Sydney, Australia.

2

CHAPTER 1

Particular Challenges in Microencapsulation of Insulin-Producing Cells for the Treatment of Diabetes Mellitus

Stéphanie Bilodeau and Jean-Pierre Hallé[*]

University of Montreal/Centre Research Hospital Maisonneuve-Rosemont Research Laboratory on Bio-artificial Therapies, 5415 boul. L'Assomption, Montreal (Quebec), H1T 2M4, Canada

Abstract: The ideal treatment for type 1 diabetes mellitus implies minute-to-minute modulations of insulin release according to the continuous variations of blood glucose. This can be accomplished by the transplantation of insulin-producing cells that are located in the pancreatic islets of Langerhans (islets). To avoid the use of potentially toxic immunosuppressive drugs, the cells may be entrapped within semi-permeable microcapsules. While several issues related to this task are similar to those found in other applications of cell microencapsulation, the present chapter emphasizes the challenges that are particular to the development of a bioartificial endocrine pancreas. In contrast to monocellular preparations used in other applications, islets are well organized cell cluster comprising 1500-3000 cells. However, the microcapsule membrane prevents transplanted islets from being re-vascularised. Therefore, oxygen supply depends upon diffusion only. Oxygen has to travel a relatively long distance to reach the cells located in the center of encapsulated islets. Central necrosis occurs, particularly in the largest islets. In contrast, dispersed single islet cells are very resistant to hypoxia but cannot function properly since they require cell-to-cell interactions. Thus, oxygen supply to encapsulated islet cells is crucial. Other issues that are particular to the bioartificial endocrine pancreas involve the number of islets to be transplanted, the rapid response of insulin release to variations of blood glucose levels, the limited supply of allogeneic islets from deceased donors and the implantation site. This chapter addresses all of these issues, as well as promising strategies that are being explored to overcome these hurdles.

Keywords: Microencapsulation, diabetes, insulin, oxygenation, islet of Langerhans, aggregates, implantation, clinical trials, islet transplantation, bioengineering, immunosuppression, oxygen supply, hypoxia, xenografts.

1. DIABETES MELLITUS

1.1. Definition, Pathogenesis and Principal Types of Diabetes Mellitus

In the non-diabetic individual, the blood glucose level is tightly regulated and

---

*Address correspondance to Jean-Pierre Hallé:** University of Montreal/Centre Research Hospital Maisonneuve-Rosemont Research Laboratory on Bio-artificial Therapies, 5415 boul. L'Assomption, Montreal (Quebec), H1T 2M4, Canada; Tel: +1 514 252 3400; Fax: 1-514-252-3561; E-mail: hallejp@videotron.ca

maintained within a narrow normal range. A diagnosis of diabetes is made when the fasting blood glucose is $\geq$ 7.0 mM and/or the blood glucose two-hours after the ingestion of 75 g of glucose is $\geq$ 11.1 mM. The two principal types of diabetes are type 1 (T1DM), known as insulin dependent or juvenile diabetes, and type 2 (T2DM) diabetes, formerly called non-insulin dependent or adult onset diabetes. T1DM is caused by the auto-immune destruction of the insulin producing β-cells, located in the islets of Langerhans of the pancreas. T2DM is caused by a combination of resistance to the action of insulin and a relative decrease of insulin secretion.

Currently, research on β-cell replacement aims at developing a treatment for T1DM. However, it cannot be excluded that similar approaches will eventually be used for T2DM, in combination with treatments that target other defects found in this complex disease. The use of allogeneic islets from deceased donors would provide enough islets for $\leq$ 1% of potential T1DM recipients. As long as this is the only source of islets for human application, it is unlikely that the treatment will be extended to T2DM. Nevertheless, if other methods are developed, such as the production of efficient insulin-producing cells from stem/progenitor cells and an unlimited supply of cells thus becomes available, other indications, including T2DM, would probably be considered.

1.2. Long Term Complications are Severe and Related to Poor Blood Glucose Control

When diabetes is poorly controlled, chronic hyperglycaemia leads to devastating complications, such as nephropathy, retinopathy, neuropathy, coronary artery disease, stroke, peripheral artery insufficiency and amputations. There is a correlation between poor metabolic control and the development of neurological, micro vascular and macro vascular complications of diabetes [1, 2]. Moreover, it has been shown that improving blood glucose control, using intensive insulin therapy, delays these complications [3, 4] .

1.3. Current Treatment for Type 1 Diabetes: Insulin Therapy

The current treatment for T1DM is intensive insulin therapy. Patients measure their blood glucose levels by pricking their fingers, ideally at least four times a day. They use this information to adjust the doses of their insulin injections that are taken four times a day, *i.e.* fast acting insulin before each meal and long-acting insulin that can be given at bedtime or in the morning. For the decisions regarding the insulin doses, they also take into account the amount of physical activity (recent and anticipated), the anticipated food intake (carbohydrate counting for adjusting the fast acting insulin doses), stress, menstrual cycle, seasons, intercurrent diseases, *etc.*

In the non diabetic individual, the amount of insulin that is produced by the β-cells and released into the bloodstream is continuously and precisely modulated depending upon the current blood glucose and the variations during the preceding minutes. This is the only way to achieve the complete normalization of the 24 hour blood glucose profile. Insulin therapy does not provide as precise and accurate blood glucose levels as the physiological regulation. The patient himself makes decisions regarding insulin doses depending upon the results of self monitoring of blood glucose (finger pricking), and blood glucose is not precisely regulated every minute.

1.4. Non-Encapsulated Biological Transplantation (Whole Pancreas Transplantation and Islet Transplantation)

Currently, only two emerging treatments provide a physiological control of blood glucose levels: the transplantation of the whole pancreas and the transplantation of only the endocrine (hormone secreting) part of the pancreas, *i.e.* the islets of Langerhans (islets). To date, whole pancreas transplantation has been more successful than islet transplantation in maintaining long-term insulin independence. However, this treatment requires major surgery and strong immunosuppression protocols, thus is limited to severe cases or kidney and pancreas transplantation recipients [5]. Since insulin-producing cells represent only 1-2 % of the pancreas mass, ≈ 98% of the pancreatic tissue that is transplanted is not required for β-cell replacement and is potentially immunogenic. In contrast, islet transplantation can be performed on an out-patient basis using non invasive techniques. Moreover, it raises the hope of reduced immunosuppression and potentially allows the development of methods to completely eliminate the use of immunosuppressive drugs. Whether whole pancreas or islet, these transplantations allow the modulation of insulin release according to the blood glucose levels 1440 minutes a day, 365 days a year. This is a requirement for optimal diabetes control but for no other disease.

1.5. Encapsulated Islet Transplantation

In order to avoid the requirement for immunosuppression, cells to be transplanted should be physically protected from the recipient immune system using semipermeable membranes. Three geometric configurations have been experimented: intra-vascular devices, extra vascular macrocapsules and extra vascular microcapsules. The transplantation of microencapsulated islets has normalized the blood glucose, without immunosuppression, in different animal models of diabetes. In the 1980s and 1990s, a majority of the research on encapsulated cell transplantation has been conducted for application to the treatment of diabetes. This review is focused on the microencapsulation of islets for the treatment of insulin dependent diabetes.

2. NON-ENCAPSULATED ISLET TRANSPLANTATION

2.1. Development of Islet Transplantation Towards Clinical Application

Islet transplantation is a promising treatment that allows minute-to-minute adjustment of insulin release and considerable improvement of blood glucose control. Continuous progress has been achieved over the last few decades by several research groups on different aspects of this therapeutic approach. In the 1970s, Ballinger and Lacey [6] first succeeded to transplant isolated islets into diabetic rodents. To translate this method into large animal models and humans has been a difficult task. One of the first successful transplantations in humans was performed in 1990 in Pittsburg. This group reported the induction of insulin independence in 50% of recipients with non auto-immune diabetes, but the islet response to glucose was not optimal [7]. The success rate in patients with type 1 diabetes has remained low until 2000. According to the 2001 International Islet Transplant Registry [8], from 1990 to 1999, only 11 % of recipients maintained insulin independence at one year post transplant. In 2000, the Edmonton group reported that 7 successive patients with type 1 diabetes had achieved insulin independence following islet transplantation [9]. The "Edmonton protocol" included several modifications of the standard procedure, such as a nondiabetogenic immunosuppression regimen, the use of fresh islets, careful pancreas and recipient selection and an adequate number of islets (> 11,000 islet equivalents/kg recipient body weight). The Edmonton group has now succeeded to induce insulin independence in over 100 patients. A multicenter study, "the International Islet Transplantation Trial" [10] , has been conducted as an attempt to generalize the Edmonton method. Nevertheless, a limited number of centers were able to achieve similar results. Moreover, whereas initial studies showed better results when pancreas sampling, islet isolation and transplantation were performed at the same center, recent data support collaboration between centers that are located as much as 800 kilometers apart. These improved results could be achieved because of technical ameliorations of the preservation and transport of the total pancreas and isolated islets as well as standardization of pancreas procurement procedures. An international group, *the Swiss-French GRAGIL (Groupe de Recherche sur la Greffe d'Îlots de Langerhans) network,* is a collaboration of many European hospitals for the distribution of compatible isolated islets to be transplanted across Switzerland and France.

2.2. Benefits of Clinical Islet Transplantation

The Edmonton group first reported the induction of insulin independence in 100% of seven consecutive recipients with type 1 diabetes. Nevertheless, insulin treatment has to be re-introduced in several patients, after a median time of 15 months [11]. Insulin independence is only one of several benefits for the recipients of islet transplantation. Other objectives are important as well. Even patients that have to resume certain form of insulin therapy (usually at lower doses than before transplantation), or could not initially withdraw insulin completely, have benefited from the procedure. The avoidance of needles is only a small part of patient's relief. Increased flexibility and liberty regarding several aspects of daily life is considerably improved after transplantation. Most of transplanted patients have been selected because of poorly controlled diabetes, frequent or severe hypoglycemia and/or hypoglycemia unawareness. Following transplantation, hemoglobin A1C and premeal blood glucose are normal or close to normal. Those who had hypoglycemia unawareness have recovered normal perception of hypoglycemia. Hopefully, with longer follow-up, larger patient cohorts and improved technology, these treatments may prove to prevent long-term diabetes complications. It must be emphasized that the benefits that are described above occur only in patients with a persisting graft function as demonstrated by C-peptide levels.

2.3. Limitations of Non-Encapsulated Islet Transplantation

2.3.1. Immunosuppression

The most important limitation of islet transplantation is the requirement for life-long immunosuppression. Such treatments decrease the immune defence against infections and cancers. Severe and opportunistic infections or cancers are relatively rare in patients undergoing the immunosuppression protocols that are used for islet transplant [12]. Nonetheless, when they occur, they may be life threatening. Moreover, some immunosuppressors have direct toxicity on the kidney and liver, may deteriorate the lipid profile and induce hypertension [12, 13]. Thus, immunosuppressors may negatively counterbalance the positive effects of improved blood glucose control on renal and cardiovascular complications. For such risks to be acceptable, clear advantages of the approach over current treatments must be demonstrated. Furthermore, when islets are transplanted into the liver (the currently preferred implantation site), oral administration of these drugs may have a direct toxic effect on islets [14] and contribute to the limited islet survival. This results from the fact that the intestinal veins drain into the portal circulation. Finally, the follow-up of immunosuppressed patients is labour intensive for the patient as well as the medical team.

2.3.2. Loss of β-Cells Mass

It has been shown that there is a massive β-cell loss in the early post-transplant period. Factors that are potentially involved include low oxygen supply, nutrient deprivation and unspecific inflammatory reactions [15, 16]. It has been estimated that 50% of the β-cell mass is lost within the 15 first days [17]. The possible immunological reasons for the graft failure are chronic allogeneic rejection, recurrence of autoimmunity and β-cell toxicity due to the immunosuppressive treatment [18]. Also, the inflammatory reaction affects the graft function and leads to early islet cell loss. Macrophages release cytokines that are involved in the dysfunction and death of islet cells, such as interleukin-1β (IL-1β), tumour necrosis factor-α (TNF-α) and interferon-γ (IFN-γ). Nitric oxide (NO), prostaglandins (PGs) and reactive oxygen species (ROS) are also secreted and are harmful for islets [15]. Indeed, macrophage depletion immediately before transplantation was shown to improve islet cell survival [19]. This loss of β-cells may lead to early graft failure.

Non-immunological factors also explain early graft failure. The islet isolation procedure is stressful. Islets are exposed to ischemia during isolation, which decreases the yield, quality and survival of islet cells [20]. Also, the collagenase used for pancreas digestion destroys the extracellular matrix (ECM). The ECM is composed of proteins surrounding islets and is implicated in many cellular processes, such as proliferation, differentiation, migration, apoptosis, etc. The ECM destruction leads to central necrosis and apoptosis [21-23]. Furthermore, the loss of tropic stimuli that are provided by exocrine pancreas elements increases the problematic [24]. Another important problem is that blood vessels are disrupted from the rest of the vasculature.

The massive β-cells loss leads to two important consequences: the requirement for more than one donor and the high rate of recurrence of insulin dependence. Indeed, two to four donors or pancreases per recipient are required for achieving insulin independence [9]. A striking observation is the large mass of islets that is required to induce insulin independence. The normal pancreas contains approximately one million islets. It has been shown that ≈ 90 % of the pancreas must be destroyed to induce diabetes in the absence of insulin resistance. Therefore, theoretically, slightly more than 100,000 islets should be enough to reverse diabetes. Approximately 800,000 islets per recipient have actually been required to achieve this objective (15,000 islet equivalents/kg of recipient body weight). Furthermore, following such transplantations, the blood glucose response to a meal challenge is considerably improved but the insulin response is only about 20% of that seen in normal individual, revealing very low reserves [12]. Considering that the normal pancreas contains enough islets for treating several recipients, these observations reflect the loss of a large number of islets during the different steps of the procedure.

Another concern is the high rate of recurrence of insulin dependence. Considering the limited β-cell reserve that was observed immediately after transplantation, this was not unexpected. However, it is somehow disappointing to see recurrence rates of 40% and 90% at one year and 5 years post-transplantation, respectively [11]. This indicates a loss of islets after transplantation as well.

3. MICROENCAPSULATED ISLET TRANSPLANTATION: OVERVIEW AND PROGRESS

Microencapsulation is a promising solution to avoid the requirement for immunosuppression. Islets are entrapped within a semi-permeable membrane, which allows the diffusion of small molecules, such as insulin, glucose and oxygen but prevents the contact between the transplanted cells and the larger cells and antibodies of the immune system. The islet cells ensure a fine regulation of blood glucose while the microcapsules protect them from immune damage. Thus, the main advantage of microencapsulation is to eliminate the need for toxic immunosuppressive treatment. Furthermore, the membrane protection may permit the transplantation of non human donor islets (xenograft, stem/progenitor or bioengineered cells), as a potential solution for the limited supply of cadaveric human islets.

The microencapsulation of islets in alginate-poly-L-lysine microcapsules was first described by Lim and Sun [25] and it is still the most common microencapsulation method. In their first publication in 1980, they showed that implantation of microencapsulated islets could restore normoglycemia for 2-3 weeks in streptozotocin-induced diabetic rats, as compared to only 6 to 8 days with non-encapsulated islets. The first implantations in a large animal model were achieved in 1992 and were successful for 7 to 24 weeks [26]. The first allotransplantations of encapsulated tissue in human was experimented with pancreatic islets and parathyroid cells in the 1990's [27, 28]. The encapsulated islet experiment was performed using islets from 8 donors and what was described as a sub-immunosuppressive corticosteroid dose. Insulin-independence was not achieved, but a functional graft was demonstrated and glucose control was improved, using a reduced insulin dose. Parathyroid cell transplantation succeeded for at least 12 weeks, without immunosuppression. Recently, allotransplantation of encapsulated islets in humans was performed in Italy. Insulin-independence was not achieved, but blood glucose control was improved using approximately 1/3 of the previous insulin dose after transplantation of encapsulated islets from a single donor [29].

3.1. Microencapsulation Techniques

The most popular materials for encapsulating cells are alginate[28], agarose [30] , cellulose sulphate [31, 32], chitosan [33], polyhydroxyethylmetacrylate-methyl methacrylate (HEMA-MMA) [34], copolymers of acrylonitrile (AN69) [35] and polyethylene glycol (PEG) [36]. Hydrogels are the most popular because they are relatively biocompatible. Their hydrophilic nature minimizes protein and cell adhesion. They are also soft and pliable, which reduces the mechanical and frictional irritation of surrounding tissues. The most studied hydrogel is alginate, because it jellifies under physiological conditions that do not interfere with cell function [37]. This natural polymer is extracted in industrial amounts from algae. It is also produced by certain bacteria, such as *pseudomomas aeruginosa* and *azotobacter vinelandii* [38]. Alginate is composed of linear blocks of oligomers of 1-4 linked β-D-mannuronic (M) and α-L-guluronic (G) acid. It is composed of GG, MG or MM blocks of various length and proportions, depending upon the species of algae and what part of the plant it is extracted from.

Several techniques are used to encapsulate cells, depending upon the polymer that is selected and the application it is developed for. In the case of alginate, the cells are suspended in soluble sodium alginate and then entrapped in microdroplets. The droplets are transformed in gel beads when the alginate carboxyl groups cross-link with divalent cations, most commonly calcium or barium. Different techniques are used to pull the tiny droplets out of a needle, including air jet or vibration. There is also the emulsion technique for droplet fabrication. The use of an electrostatic pulse generator allows the production of smaller microcapsules. The microcapsule size was decreased from 800 μm to 185 μm diameters using this technique [39-41]. Reducing the microcapsule size improves the ability of oxygen to diffuse up to the islet cells. A potential pitfall is that smaller microcapsules are associated with more bulging of islets out of the capsule surface, which may increase the immunogenicity of the transplant [42].

It is also common to coat alginate beads with a polycation, which binds to negatively charged alginate molecules. The most commonly used polycations are poly-L-Lysine (PLL), poly-L-Ornithine (PLO), poly-D-Lysine and polymethylene-co-guanidine. This procedure has several advantages, such as increasing the mechanical stability of the microcapsule, allowing the control of the membrane porosity and preventing the beads from being dissolved by physiological chelator agents. However, soluble and non-complexed PLL has been shown to be an inflammatory molecule, which leads to fibrotic overgrowth when it is not properly bound to alginate [43, 44] and it may decrease encapsulated cell viability if use in too high concentrations. Therefore, some research groups have selected to use non PLL coated alginate beads. In this case, calcium is usually replaced by barium, as gelling divalent cations. Barium has a higher affinity for alginate than calcium [45] and allows to make stronger beads without using PLL. Another approach is to develop techniques to improve the neutralisation of PLL reactive residues. More research is needed to optimize this aspect of the method. This includes the development of new polymers for the outer coating of alginate-polycation microcapsules.

4. SPECIFIC CHALLENGES OF MICROENCAPSULATED ISLET TRANSPLANTATION: OXYGEN SUPPLY TO MICROENCAPSULATED ISLETS

Other chapters of this eBook address different issues related to the microencapsulation of all types of cells. The present chapter emphasizes the challenges that are specific to the bioartificial endocrine pancreas. Islets have a particular physiology leading to different challenges. In contrast to monocellular preparations used in other applications, islets are cell clusters. They have a high oxygen demand and they are physiologically well vascularized. Necrosis of cells that are located in the center of islets has been observed, affecting particularly the largest islets. This phenomenon has been explained by the longer distance that oxygen has to travel to reach these cells. This fact is thought to play an important role in early and late graft failure. Therefore, the most important particular challenge in islet encapsulation is the oxygenation of islet cells. A brief description of relevant anatomic and physiological features of the islets as well as the biological effects of hypoxia on cells will precede the discussion of the challenges of islet transplantation, non-encapsulated and encapsulated.

4.1. Islet Physiology

4.1.1. Multicellular Structures

Pancreatic islets are spheroid structures that contain approximately 1500-3000 cells. They have a mean diameter of 150 μm, with a range varying between 50 and 500 μm [46, 47]. The average human pancreas contains between 300 000 and 1 500 000 islets. The islet mass represents only 1-2% of the total pancreatic mass. The pancreas is composed of islets (hormone secreting cells), acinar cells (digestive enzyme secreting cells) and ducts (duct cells secrete mainly $NaHCO_3$ and some peptides, such as IGF-II and NGF [24]). Islets are composed of endocrine (hormone releasing) cells and endothelial cells.

4.1.2. Islet Endocrine Cells: Their Respective Roles and Interactions

The islets of Langerhans contain at least 5 different types of endocrine cells, α, β, δ, PP and ε, which secrete respectively glucagon, insulin, somatostatin, polypeptide P and ghrelin. β-cells secrete amylin as well, in a 1:100 amylin/insulin ratio. Human islets are composed of 60% β-cells, 30% α-cells, less than 10% δ-cells and less than 5% PP and ε cells [48]. Whereas insulin is the major player for blood glucose regulation, each of these hormones has a specific role in the carbohydrate metabolism. When β-cells detect higher blood glucose, they secrete insulin into the bloodstream. Islets contain β-cells with different thresholds for triggering insulin secretion; thus as blood glucose increases, a larger number of β-cells release insulin, resulting in higher blood insulin levels. Insulin travels through the whole body, binds to insulin receptors in insulin responsive tissues and activates different intracellular signaling pathways. Insulin mechanisms of action include the production and translocation to the cell membrane of glucose transporters which facilitates glucose entry into the target cell. Glucagon is secreted when the blood glucose is low. It activates neoglucogenesis and glycogenolysis, increasing hepatic glucose production. Somatostatin is an inhibitory hormone; it suppresses the secretion of pancreatic and digestive hormones. The exact role of polypeptide P is unknown and ghrelin has a role in hunger. In rodents, islets have a specific architecture: β-cells are located in the center while the other types of cells are at the periphery (Fig. **1**) [49]. However, this organization is not the same in human islets, which have a random cell distribution [48, 50].

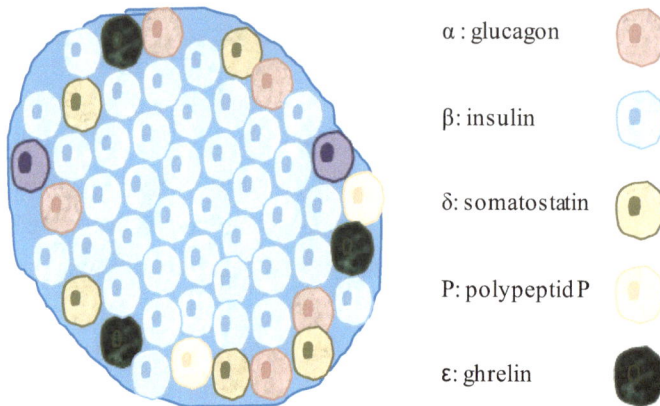

Figure 1: Islets of Langerhans are composed of 5 different cell types, α, β, δ, P, ε, secreting each a specific hormone, respectively glucagon, insulin, somatostatin, polypeptid P and ghrelin. In rodents, β-cells are located in the center while the other types of cells are at the periphery.

Islet cell-to-cell contacts are essential for β-cell differentiation and function [51-53]. Indeed, dispersed single islet cells have a poor insulin secretion and they do not respond to glucose [53, 54]. Islet cells interact *via* gap junctions composed of protein connexin-36 [55] allowing cells to communicate and coordinate their response. Calcium-dependent adhesion molecules (CAM), such as E-cadherins (epithelial-cadherin) and NCAM (neural-CAM), are also responsible for cell-to-cell contacts and interactions [56, 57]. They regulate the aggregation of islet cells and maintain the primary islet architecture [56-58]. E-cadherins influence islet function and proliferation as well [59-61].

4.1.2. Islet Vascularisation in the Native Pancreas

Islets are highly vascularised structures [50, 62]. They receive 10-20% of the total blood flow through the pancreas, although they represent 1-2% of its mass [63-65]. This assures islets to meet their high metabolic demand. Islet vasculature is a highly specialised glomerular-like structure. Small arterioles enter into the core of the islets and a network of capillaries drains into venules to carry the blood to the periphery. Capillary endothelia are highly fenestrated [66], which accelerates the hormone entry into the bloodstream. It is estimated that approximately 20% of insulin is delivered through this pathway, ensuring rapid insulin response to glucose increase. There are about 1500 capillaries/cm^2 in islets. This rich vascular density ensures that each β-cell is in close proximity to endothelial cells.

4.2. Biological Effects of Hypoxia

4.2.1. Role of Oxygen in Cell Metabolism and Effect of Hypoxia

Oxygen is essential for several cell processes, especially for the production of adenosine triphosphate (ATP) by cellular respiration. In aerobic metabolism, glucose is transformed into acetyl groups by a series of oxidation-reduction reactions into the acid citric cycle. Those reactions produce 8 high-energy electrons that travel to the mitochondria electron transport chain for the oxidative phosphorylation. Electrons are used to reduce O_2 into H_2O which generates the proton gradient that is required for ATP synthesis. Moderate hypoxia switches the cell metabolism from aerobic respiration to anaerobic glycolysis. In this case, glycolysis is the process that is used by cells to generate energy. In those reactions, one molecule of glucose is metabolized into two molecules of pyruvate with the production of 2 ATP molecules. Pyruvate is then fermented into lactate to produce NADH. However, only a small fraction of energy available from complete glucose combustion is produced by this pathway [67]. Since ATP is required for many essential cellular functions, moderate oxygen deprivation may have deleterious consequences. In islets, ATP is required, amongst other things, for glucose responsive insulin secretion.

4.2.2. Severe or Prolonged Hypoxia Induces Apoptosis

The cell response to hypoxia depends upon the oxygen level. An acute or mild hypoxia leads to cell adaptation and survival response. If hypoxia persists or if it is more severe, the cells enter in apoptosis. Apoptosis or "programmed cell death" prevents propagation of deleterious effects of overgrowth, mutations, infections or cell damages. The caspase protein family has a major role in apoptosis. They are cysteine proteases activated by pro-apoptotic stimuli. Some caspases (such as -8 and -10) are initiator caspases; they cleave the effector caspases (such as -3, -10), which in turn degrade intracellular protein substrates. This induces the classical apoptosis morphological changes, such as chromatin condensation, nuclear degeneration and cellular dehydration [68].

There are two major apoptotic pathways, one activated by extracellular events (extrinsic pathway) and one activated by intracellular events (intrinsic pathway). The first one may be mediated by inflammatory cytokines or triggered by direct cytotoxic lymphocytes-T engagement. It activates caspase pathways [68, 69]. The intrinsic pathway is induced by DNA damage, hypoxia, nutrient deprivation, ROS, *etc.* They activate the Bcl-2 mitochondrial pathway. There are two classes of Bcl-2 protein: pro-apoptotic (such as Bim, Bid, Bax…) and anti-apoptotic Bcl-2 proteins (such as Bcl-2 and Bcl-xl). There is an important balance between the two types of signals. Apoptosis is triggered when pro-apoptotic protein concentrations are higher than the anti-apoptotic ones. When cells receive a pro-apoptotic signal, pro-apoptotic Bcl-2 proteins are activated and translocated into the mitochondria. They bind and inactivate anti-apoptotic proteins. They form a pore in the mitochondrial membrane inducing the release of cytochrome c into the cytosol, which complexes with pro-caspase-9 and Apaf-1 to form the apoptosome activating caspase-3 [70].

4.2.3. General Cell Response to Hypoxia

When cells are deprived of oxygen, they induce the transcription of genes that regulate their adaptation to low oxygen concentrations. This induction is mainly due to the activation of the hypoxia inducible factor-1 (HIF-1), a transcription factor. HIF-1 regulates cell survival under hypoxic conditions. It is a heterodimeric basic helix-loop-helix transcription factor composed of HIF-1α and HIF-1β, an aryl hydrocarbon receptor nuclear translocator (ARNT) [71]. The latter is constitutively expressed, whereas HIF-1α is activated in hypoxic conditions. In normoxic conditions, two HIF-1α proline residues are hydroxylated by a family of iron(II)-dependent prolyl-hydroxylase. It binds to von Hippel Lindau protein (vHL), it is polyubiquitinated and degraded by the proteasome [72, 73]. When cells detect a low oxygen concentration, it inhibits the prolyl-hydroxylase, HIF-1α is stabilized, translocated to the nucleus, it dimerizes with HIF-1β and HIF-1 is activated. It binds to genes that contain hypoxia response elements (HREs) in their transcriptional promoters and it leads to the induction of genes implicated in the adaptation to hypoxia, modulation of angiogenesis, oxygen transport, iron metabolism, glycolysis, glucose uptake, growth factor signaling, apoptosis and metastasis (Fig. **2**) [74]. For example, some of those genes can promote cell survival by increasing oxygen delivery to hypoxic tissues (erythropoietin), inducing revascularization (VEGF) or increasing glucose transport (Glut-1) and glycolytic enzymes (lactate deshydrogenase A).

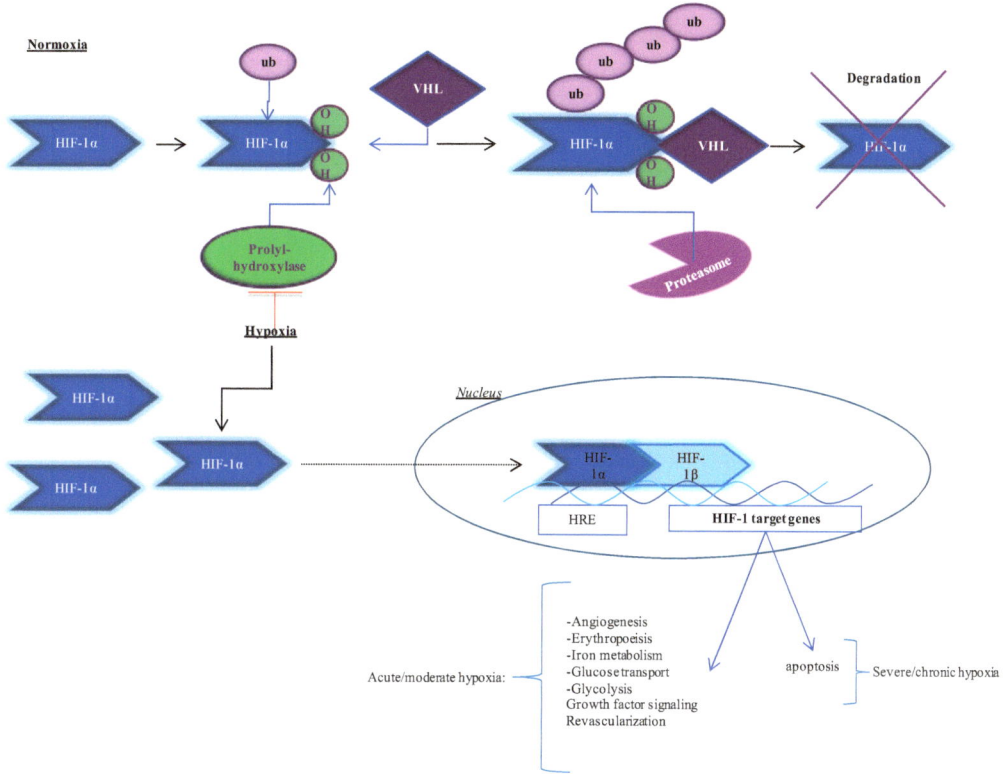

Figure 2: Hypoxia activation of HIF-1. In normal oxygen concentration, HIF-1α is hydroxylated by a prolyl-hydroxylase, Von Hippel Lindau protein binds it; then it is ubiquitinated and degraded by the proteasome. In hypoxia, the prolyl-hydroxylase is inhibited, HIF-1α goes into the nucleus and binds to HIF-1β to form the active transcription factor. It binds the Hypoxia Response Element and activates transcription of target genes that are implicated in angiogenesis, erythropoesis or apoptosis.

There are three isoforms of HIF: HIF-1α, HIF-2α/endothelial PAS domain protein (EPAS) and HIF-3α. Despite similar structures, they have different activation mechanisms, tissue distribution and target genes [75]. HIF-1α is more sensitive to O_2 concentration variations, while HIF-2α mediates a survival response to O_2–independent variations, such as growth factors, cytokines and hypoglycaemia [76]. HIF-3α may be a modulator of hypoxic gene induction [77].

HIF-1α is expressed as a protective hypoxia factor. Under moderate hypoxia, HIF-1α induces anti-apoptotic pathways, such as IAP-2 [78]. However, if hypoxia persists or if it is severe, the protective response fails and the cells enter into hypoxia-mediated apoptosis. HIF-1 induces apoptosis *via* BNIP3, a Bcl-2 family protein. The BNIP3 gene promoter has a functional HRE [79]. Indeed, HIF-1α knocked-out cells do not undergo hypoxia-mediated apoptosis [80]. HIF-1 has an important role in hypoxia response and in the balance between cell survival and cell death during hypoxia.

4.2.4. Islet Cell Response to Hypoxia

As mentioned earlier, hypoxia has a negative effect on cellular functions that require high cellular ATP concentrations. In islets, insulin secretion is ATP-dependent. Indeed, moderate hypoxia leads to a 50% decrease in glucose stimulated insulin secretion [81]. However, basal secretion is less affected, because this process requires lower amounts of ATP [82]. HIF-1α was shown to be strongly expressed in non encapsulated transplanted islets during the 14 days following their transplantation. It was correlated with a decrease in insulin secretion, and increase of β-cell death. HIF-1α expression decreases as revascularization progresses [83]. Severe hypoxia has also been shown to lead to β-cell death, due to necrosis and apoptosis [83, 84]. After only six hours in hypoxia, islets may show nuclear pyknosis and caspase-3 expression due to activation of HIF-α1 and BNIP3 [85].

Another mediator of hypoxic injuries is AMP-activated protein kinase (AMPK). It was shown to be activated by hypoxia in non encapsulated islets. It activates caspase-3 and it generates reactive oxygen species (ROS) [86] which damage cellular proteins, membrane lipids and nucleic acids. Hypoxia also induces biochemical reactions that lead to ROS production and cause cell death. Antioxidant treatments have been applied to isolated islets and were shown to increase islet cell viability and function [87].

In encapsulated islets, hypoxia was also associated with a loss of islet function and viability. Furthermore, some harmful proteins have been shown to be expressed in islets in the presence of low O_2 concentration, such as inducible nitric oxide synthase (iNOS) and monocyte chemoattractant protein-1 (MCP-1) [82, 88]. iNOS expression might be induced by HIF-1 and is responsible for nitric oxide (NO) production. NO is a short-lived free radical that causes cell damages and death by inducing DNA strand breaks [89]. Furthermore, in pancreatic β-cells, NO can inhibit insulin secretion [90]. MCP-1 attracts cytokine-producing macrophages, monocytes, memory T lymphocytes and natural killer cells [91]. All of these cells are involved in the immune reaction against microcapsules and might be toxic for islets (Fig. **3**).

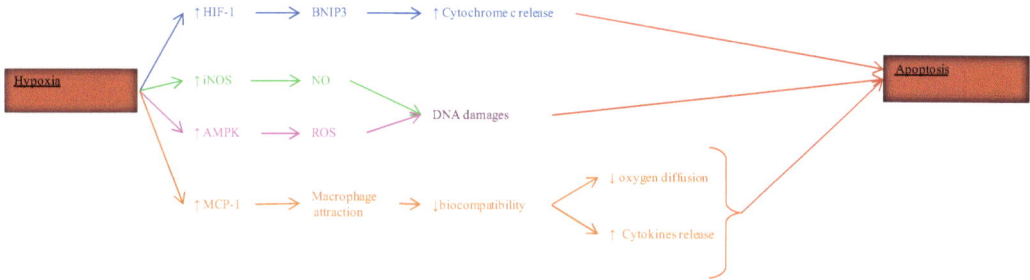

Figure 3: Hypoxia leads to apoptosis *via* different pathways.

4.3. Oxygenation Challenges in Non-Encapsulated Islet Transplantation

4.3.1. Transplantation Site

One important factor in non-encapsulated islet oxygenation is the transplantation site and its oxygen partial pressure (pO_2). Firstly, oxygen is transported into the blood by red blood cell haemoglobin in concentrations varying between 100 mmHg and 40 mmHg. Haemoglobin binds oxygen and ejects carbon dioxide in the lungs by diffusion. The blood is distributed throughout different organs and haemoglobin exchanges oxygen for tissue carbon dioxide. The haemoglobin-oxygen dissociation curve is such that the affinity of haemoglobin for oxygen is high at the pH found in the lung and low in periphery.

Oxygen tension varies within and between organs in function of their vascularisation and oxygen consumption rates. Within native pancreatic islets, because they are well vascularised, the mean pO_2 is around 40 mmHg. In the kidney cortex, the spleen and the liver, the most common transplantation sites for non encapsulated islets, oxygen tension is near 15 mmHg, 30 mmHg and 5 mmHg, respectively [92]. When transplanted into the kidney cortex, the liver and the spleen, islet oxygen concentration is similar, between 5-10 mmHg O_2 (1% O_2), although the three organs have different pO_2 tensions [92]. The oxygen tension that is measured in transplanted islets is only a fraction of the tension found in native islets [92-95].

4.3.2. Revascularization of Transplanted Islets

During islet isolation, islet blood vessels are disrupted from the rest of the vasculature. When non encapsulated islets are transplanted, revascularization and connexion to the host vasculature occur within 7 to 14 days after transplantation [96, 97]. An important proportion of transplanted islets die during this period and it correlates with the low oxygen supply [17]. Moreover, the decreased oxygen tension is still present after the revascularization for up to 9 months post-transplantation and the vascular density of non encapsulated islets remains diminished on long term [94, 95, 98] showing inadequate revascularization and its prolonged effect.

4.4. Oxygen Supply Challenges to Microencapsulated Islets

The problem of revascularization is even more important for encapsulated islets, because the microcapsule membrane prevents the blood vessels from reconnecting to the host vasculature. In this case, the oxygenation depends upon diffusion only. The pO_2 values are 20% lower than in non encapsulated tissues [99]. Moreover, the oxygen depleted-zone is twice larger in microencapsulated than free islets [99]. This is explained by the assumption that within microcapsules there is no convection movement. This creates an oxygen and nutrient gradient from the capsule surface to the center of the islet. The pO_2 in the middle of microencapsulated islets is 50% lower than in non encapsulated islets [100]. This is one of the major barriers to the success of microencapsulated islet transplantation [101].

Transplanted microencapsulated islets often show central necrosis, which affects particularly the largest islets. This observation suggests that oxygen does not reach the cells located in the center of these islets. In order to oxygenate encapsulated islets, oxygen diffuses from blood vessel to target cells. It has first to travel from the blood vessel to the microcapsule surface, then through the microcapsule and within the islet, in order to reach every cell, including those located in the center of islets. In most mammalian tissues, the diffusion distance between blood capillaries and each cell is limited to 150-200 μm [102, 103].

4.4.1. The Implantation Site

The implantation site is the most important factor determining the local O_2 concentration and the distance between blood vessels and the capsule surface. The peritoneum is the most common implantation site for microencapsulated islets merely because it allows enough space for a large transplant. However, it is not well vascularised. In the peritoneal cavity, the pO_2 varies between 26 and 70 mm Hg [104]. Moreover, microcapsules are in continuous motion, which induces a varying distance between the transplant and the blood vessels. In that situation, depending upon their exact location, the pO_2 may fall close to 0% [105].

4.4.2. Oxygen Diffusion

Other limitations to oxygen transport include those related to oxygen diffusion within microcapsules and islets. The microcapsule size is an important parameter for this issue. Standard microcapsules have an average diameter of 800 μm. Using the electrostatic pulse system, we are routinely producing microcapsules of an average size of 300-350 μm diameter [106-108]. Even with this system, to reach cells located in the islet center, oxygen has to travel 175 μm plus the distance between the blood vessel and the capsule. The oxygenation is still limited. Smaller capsules would be useful from an oxygenation perspective but they risk increasing the protrusion of islets out of the capsule surface.

4.4.3. Size of Islets

Another important parameter is the size of islets. The average islet diameter is 150 μm with a range of 50 to 400 μm. Smaller islets have been shown to provide more insulin and experience better survival both in normoxic and hypoxic culture and have been more predictive of clinical islet transplantation efficiency [109, 110]. It has also been predicted that as much as 25% of the volume of a 200 μm diameter islet is below the critical oxygen threshold, *i.e.* the point at which cells die from necrosis if maintained for a sufficient time. This is compared to 5% and 0% for islets of 150 and 100 μm diameter, respectively [111]. Furthermore, there are gradients of oxygen partial pressure within isolated islets, with a difference of 40 mmHg between the surface and the center of the islet. This gradient increases as islet diameter is larger [99]. Other factors include the cell density of the implant and its geometrical characteristics [101]. A huge amount of cells in a small volume decreases the ability of oxygen to diffuse freely. The surface/volume ratio has to be high to allow access of oxygen to more cells.

4.4.4. Biocompatibility

Microcapsule immunogenicity is also an important factor because an immune response to the implant is almost always associated with graft failure [100, 112]. For example, when islets were encapsulated using non purified alginate, a non-specific foreign body reaction has occurred against microcapsules. This pericapsular cell overgrowth is initially composed principally of activated macrophages, followed by fibroblasts and extracellular matrix deposition. The inflammatory cells that adhere to the capsule surface secrete small cytokines, chemokines and free radicals, which may cross the capsule membrane and damage encapsulated cells. Moreover, pericapsular fibrosis impairs the diffusion of oxygen and nutrients. These phenomena may lead to graft failure. This pericapsular reaction has been attributed in part to alginate contaminants, such as polyphenols, endotoxins and proteins [113, 114]. Alginate purification has been shown to considerably decrease the microcapsule immunogenicity [106, 115-120]. By optimizing alginate purity and composition, alginate beads have been produced that induce less than 10% overgrowth at 12 months post peritoneal implantation [115]. Nonetheless, the lack of standardization of biomaterials and purification methods and wide variations of duration of encapsulated cell survival remains a problem (Fig. **4**).

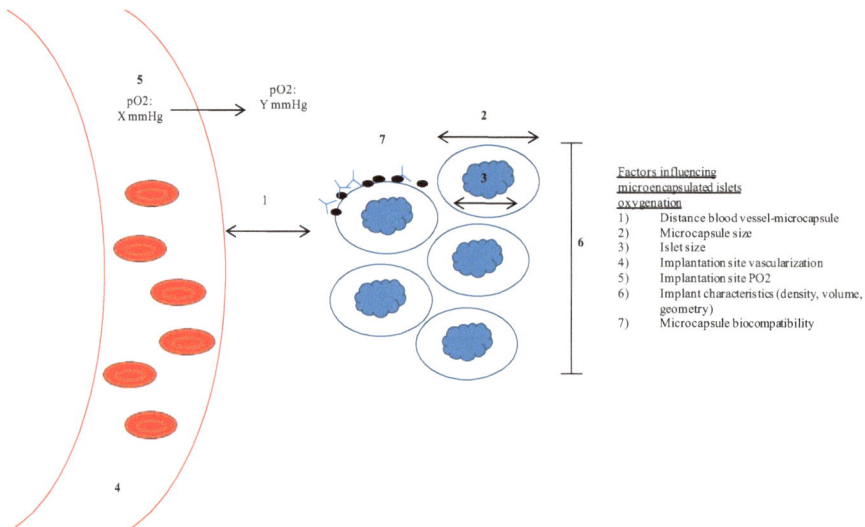

Figure 4: Several factors influencing microencapsulated islet oxygenation are illustrated in this figure: 1) Distance blood vessel-microcapsule 2) Microcapsule size; 3) Islet size; 4) Implantation site vascularization; 5) Implantation site pO$_2$; 6) Implant characteristics (density, volume, geometry); 7) Microcapsule biocompatibility.

There are three different immune responses against microencapsulated islets. A non-specific response due to the surgical procedure [121], the foreign body reaction against the capsule and the response provoked by the encapsulated cells, which release cytokines. Even in the absence of pericapsular overgrowth, a graft failure may occur after an average of 6 to 20 weeks post-transplantation [115]. It has been shown that when islets are exposed to interleukin-1β (IL-1β) and tumour necrosis factor-α (TNF-α), which are released by macrophages, they secrete cytokines, such as monocyte chemoattractant protein-1 (MCP-1), macrophage inflammatory protein (MIP), nitric oxide (NO) and interleukine-6 (IL-6). These cytokines attract and activate more inflammatory cells and this process results in a vicious cycle [122, 123]. Although the microcapsule membrane blocks the access of antibodies and immune cells to the islets, smaller molecules can penetrate into the capsule and damage the islets [124, 125].

4.5. Strategies for Improving Oxygen Supply to Encapsulated Islet Cells

Several research groups are currently investigating different approaches to improve the oxygenation of encapsulated islets. An important consequence of improved oxygen delivery to islet cells is to increase the efficiency of transplanted islets, thereby reducing the number of islets that has to be transplanted, thus the total implant volume. This section reviews the main solutions to the challenges that are presented above.

4.5.1. Transplantation Site

Firstly, the transplantation site is the main determinant of the local pO_2 concentration and the distance between blood vessels and the microcapsule surface. The development of methods to produce smaller microcapsules may allow the experimentation of alternative sites to the peritoneum. Bioartificial sites offer an interesting alternative. For example, a prevascularised expanded polytetrafluoroethylene solid support can form a hypervascularized, removable bio-artificial implantation site that could allow microencapsulated islets to be in close proximity of blood vessels [126]. Microcapsules can also be enveloped within a vascular prosthesis that is directly anastomosed to blood vessels [127]. This method provides excellent proximity to blood vessels. However, it is limited by the fact that it is a relatively small compartment and the risk of thrombosis.

This approach has thus been abandoned by most research groups. Another method is based on the use of a natural photosynthetic oxygen generator, as a thermophylic strain of the unicellular alga Chlorella. It increases islet function when islets are encapsulated in this material [128].

4.5.2. Decreasing Limitations to Oxygen Diffusion within Microcapsules and Islets

Another strategy to improve the oxygenation of encapsulated islets is to decrease the limitations to oxygen diffusion within microcapsules. A few methods have been experimented to achieve such goals. We strongly believe that smaller microcapsules allow better oxygen delivery to the cells that are located in the center of islets. As well, some researchers have incorporated oxygen transporters into the polymer that is used to make the microcapsule core (*i.e.* alginate). It is possible to incorporate perfluorocarbons (PFC), an oxygen transporter, into the microcapsule matrix to enhance transplanted islet oxygenation [129, 130]. Besides improving oxygen diffusion by altering the capsule design, it is important to enhance diffusion within the islets.

4.5.3. Improving Islet Cell Resistance to Hypoxia

An alternative strategy is to improve islet cell resistance to hypoxia. Many groups are studying different techniques to improve islet oxygenation and some of the more recent are presented below. Genes or proteins can be transfected or transduced to improve the islet oxygenation. Neuroglobin, myoglobin and cytoglobin, three proteins involve in oxygen transport, were shown to have a protective effect on islets to assure a better quality of transplanted islets [131-133]. Co-expression of anti-oxidant enzymes, such as copper/zinc superoxide dismutase (SOD), extracellular SOD, and cellular glutathione peroxidase (Gpx-1), were shown to improve the graft outcome because they reduce the free radical levels [134].

The type of islet is important for the outcome of the transplantation. For example, rat and porcine neonatal islets were shown to be more resistant to hypoxia [135, 136]. Teleofish islets (*e.g.,* tilapia) can survive and function properly in a low oxygen environment, since these fish live in waters that contain little oxygen.

Transgenic tilapia, which secrete human insulin, have been developed [137]. They could be used for transplantation, taking advantage of their high resistance to hypoxia. However, their large size (up to 5 mm diameter) [138] is a problem for microencapsulation. Nevertheless, lessons could be learned by studying the mechanisms that tilapia islets use to function with low oxygen supply. Based on these findings, gene therapy could be used to modify islets.

In combination with increasing oxygen diffusion, reduction of apoptosis would be helpful for successful islet transplantation. X-linked inhibitor of apoptosis protein (XIAP) is a potent endogenous inhibitor of apoptosis. When transduced into islet, it was shown to decrease apoptosis [139, 140]. Also, Hypoglycemia/hypoxia Inducible Mitochondrial Protein (HIMP1) can have a protective effect by reducing apoptosis [141]. Another molecule that can be used for the same purpose is endothelin, which is a potent vasoconstrictor, but also a potent mitogenic/anti-apoptotic factor. It could decrease apoptosis and improve the success of islet transplantation. However, more studies are needed to improve the knowledge of this molecule [142].

5. OTHER CHALLENGES IN THE TREATMENT OF TYPE 1 DIABETES BY MICROENCAPSULATION OF INSULIN-PRODUCING CELLS

As seen in the previous sections, to get adequate oxygen and nutrient supply is more challenging in microencapsulated islet transplantation than for other applications of microencapsulation. This section presents the other issues that must be considered for the treatment of diabetes.

5.1. Rapid Response of Insulin Release to Variations of Blood Glucose Levels

Islet cells must precisely sense blood glucose variations. Diffusion is thus necessary in both directions across the membrane. Several characteristics of the pancreas contribute to tight blood glucose control. It is unlikely that a bio-artificial organ will ever perfectly match all of the physiological processes. A perfect functioning is not necessarily requested to obtain improvements over current treatment and to impact on the development of long-term complications of diabetes. Nevertheless, good understanding of physiological processes may be useful for the design of organ replacement strategies.

Following a meal, there is a rapid increment in the blood glucose level. In order to obtain an appropriate post prandial blood glucose excursion, a rapid stimulation of the insulin secreting cells takes place, which is followed by rapid insulin secretion and delivery into the bloodstream. As islets are highly vascularised, β-cells immediately sense this increase; and, at given blood glucose levels, they release insulin that has been stored in secretion vesicles (so-called first phase insulin secretion) and at the same time, they begin to synthesize and secrete new insulin. Then, the action of insulin induces the exit of glucose from the blood compartment, and the process goes the other way around: as blood glucose level goes down, an increasing number of β-cells "switch off" and the blood insulin level decreases. This turnaround must occur rapidly to avoid hypoglycaemia. Other islet hormones may contribute for fine-tuning these adjustments. Special features of the islet vasculature facilitate such rapid response, including the high vascular density within islets, the fact that β-cells are always close to capillaries and the fenestration of the islet endothelium. Since encapsulated islets are not re-vascularized, the role of the endothelium has limited importance in this case. Another feature that is absent in the encapsulated islet is the sympathic and parasympathic innervations that modulate islet hormone production, including the cephalic phase of insulin secretion. The clinical impact of these differences between the native and bio-artificial pancreases is unknown but has to be assessed.

5.2. Microencapsulation Could Allow the Use of Xenografts, Bio-Engineered or Stem Cell-Derived Cells

One major challenge of islet transplantation research is the limited supply of islets from deceased donors. This limitation is aggravated by the fact that 2 to 4 donors per recipient are currently required to induce insulin independence and by the rate of recurrence of insulin independence [11]. New sources of insulin-producing cells must be explored to allow the bioartificial pancreas to becoming generally used. However, those possibilities require various sources of cells, such as animal origin tissue, bio-engineered cells or stem cells.

5.2.1. Xenografts

Cell xenotransplantation has revealed to be much more difficult than allotransplantation. Microencapsulated xenografts have already been conducted using neonatal pig islets or pig to primate model. However, there still are concerns related to the transplantation of animal cells into humans. On theoretical grounds, some authors have questioned the protection provided by microcapsules against xenogeneic immune reactions. This view was based on the fact that xeno-antigens are presented to the T-cell receptor by the recipient antigen-presenting cells (APCs) because the donor foreign MHC complex is not recognised, whereas allo-antigens are presented by the donor APCs. While it is obvious that the donor APCs cannot go out from the microcapsules, it was hypothesized that shedding antigens could break down to a size that allows diffusion through the microcapsule membrane, thereby triggering an immune reaction. In our perspective, this is unlikely to occur. Such shedding antigens would have to form apoptotic or necrotic vesicles (which would not cross the membrane), and travel to the draining lymph node, wherein antigen presentation takes place, without being degraded. Considering that such antigens have to be smaller than the membrane molecular weight cut-off and that only a minority of minor histocompatibility complex antigens has the capacity to elicit an immune reaction, the probability that this phenomenon creates any serious problem is low. Another concern with xenotransplantation is the possibility of zoonosis, *i.e.* transmission of a virus from animals to humans, which is rare but possible.

5.2.2. Bio-Engineered Cells

Another approach for β-cell replacement is the development of completely bio-engineered cells. The initial concept was relatively simple but the endeavour revealed to be complex. The first experiments included the transfer of the pro-insulin gene in a manner that its expression was under the control of blood glucose into cells that possessed the convertases to transform pro-insulin into insulin [143-148]. It was realized that the delay between pro-insulin synthesis and insulin release is too long for an adequate response to metabolic need. The amount of insulin that is produced has to be sufficient and the selected cells must have potential for expansion. There is now a much better understanding of the challenges that have to be met for such an endeavour and much progress has been done in resolving some issues.

5.2.3. Generation of Neo-Islets from Stem/Progenitor Cells

Finally, other methods for β-cell replacement include the development of neo-islets from stem/progenitor cells. The strategy is to understand the mechanisms of islet cell formation from non endocrine cells during embryogenesis, or experimental, pathological or physiological regeneration of the pancreas, and to use this information to induce islet cell formation from non endocrine cells. This approach comprises three requirements: 1) the possibility of considerably expanding the number of cells, 2) the trans-differentiation into insulin-producing cells and 3) the insulin secretion must be glucose responsive.

No matter which method is used for β-replacement, the transplanted cells have to be protected from the immune reaction. Even if a method is eventually developed for autologous cell transplantation, such cells will have to be protected from the auto-immune reaction of type 1 diabetes.

5.3. Implantation Sites

The role of the implantation site in oxygen supply to islets has been addressed in section 4.4. As mentioned earlier, most experiments on microencapsulated islets have used the peritoneum as the implantation site. In addition to low oxygen concentration, there are several theoretical reasons that make this site inappropriate. These include the high concentration of macrophages (≈ 85 % of peritoneal cells), the continuous motion, which imposes high mechanical stress on microcapsules, delayed insulin to glucose response and blunted post prandial stimulatory effect on insulin secretion since glucose is diluted in a larger compartment (intravascular + interstitial). Nevertheless, there has been little experimental data to support this view, because only the peritoneum could accommodate enough encapsulated islets to normalize the blood glucose of diabetic animals. Recently, Dufrane *et al.* have used a simple strategy to compare the peritoneum, the kidney capsule and the subcutaneous space as implantation sites [105]. They confirmed that the peritoneum was worse than the two other sites for islet cell survival and maintenance of the capsule integrity. Thus, other implantation sites must be experimented for encapsulated islets, including the development of a bioartificial, hyper vascularised, removable, implantation site.

6. FUTURE OF ENCAPSULATED ISLET TRANSPLANTATION; CLINICAL TRIALS AND BEYOND

The microencapsulation of islets to allow their transplantation without immunosuppression has been experimented for 30 years. The fact that clinical application is lagging behind initial expectations is disappointing and has led to pessimistic views regarding the potential of this approach. In biomedical research, such a 30 years delay between the first experimentation of a new concept and clinical application is the rule rather than the exception. In the case of microencapsulation, the simplicity of the concept, great potential for application, overoptimistic views and unrealistic promises by some biotech have led scientists to underestimate the complexity of the endeavour. Pressure is exerted on researchers to accelerate the initiation of clinical trials. Others suggest that it is time for proof of concept trials in primate models. Nevertheless, we believe that experimenting in the primate model is not necessarily the best strategy at this moment (except for research in xenotransplantation). Several issues must be resolved before useful clinical trials begin. A small number of these issues require a large animal model. Nonetheless, for many research questions, using a large animal model would be thousand fold more expensive without any advantages over rodent experiments. For clinical application, the first step is to confirm the safety of microcapsules in humans, using allotransplantation. The use of primate is required only to explore xenotransplantation, which is away down the road.

What are the requirements before clinical transplantation is considered? First, biocompatibility issues have to be resolved. The immunogenicity of biomaterials, empty microcapsules and islet-containing microcapsules must be improved. Most importantly, there is a need for the standardization of biomaterials, purification procedures, *in vitro* and *in vivo* assays to assess biomaterials as well as the final product immunogenicity and bioperformance. More research should be conducted in order to improve our understanding of the microcapsule physicochemical structure at the micrometric and nanometric scale, as well as the mechanisms of the immune reaction against microcapsules. The mechanisms of the protection provided by microcapsules against the hostile environment of the recipient must also be investigated.

The proposed methods should be shown to work in animal models using a number of islet equivalents (per weight of recipient) that is applicable in humans. Efficient up-scaling methods should be developed. Several techniques that are performed manually for rodents would be too cumbersome to be done the same way for large animals or humans. Long preparation periods would result in extremely high cost and in low bioperformance of the transplant, particularly because of decreased cell viability. In the past, the clinical application of (free) islet transplantation has been possible because Ricordi and colleagues have developed a method for the automated digestion and isolation of islets [149]. Similarly, automated methods should be developed and validated for the fabrication and processing of microcapsules. This includes large-scale production of alginate beads and automated methods for coating alginate beads by polycation if required. For rodents, empty or inadequate microcapsules may be discarded by handpicking, a method that must be automated for large scale production. The capacity to produce islet/cell-containing microcapsules in a GMP (good manufacturing practice) environment is another requirement that is reinforced by regulatory agency rules. When the transplantation is performed in centers that are remote from the islet isolation and microencapsulation laboratories, proper methods for transplant storage and transport must be developed. Such development includes adequate demonstration of islet survival within microcapsules in a frozen state. Finally, the optimal transplantation site should be determined.

When clinical microencapsulated islet transplantation will be successful, several areas of research will continue to be relevant for the continuous progress of the technology. An important issue that will remain active is the development of methods to promote long-term islet survival and to allow replacement of the initial transplant when it becomes exhausted. For example, an eventual bioartificial, hypervasculazised, removable implantation site could be replenishable or replaceable. Another permanent challenge is the continuous search for alternative source of insulin-producing cells (other than allo-islets from deceased donors). This includes islets from animal origin (xenotransplantation), completely bio-engineered insulin producing cells or insulin-producing cells derived from stem/progenitor cells. Finally, clinical trials will compare the impact on the development of late diabetes complications of different treatment strategies. Such early interventions have been shown to have more impact on the prevention of complications [3].

ACKNOWLEDGEMENTS

We thank Susan K. Tam for revising the manuscript. SB has received student scholarships from Diabète Québec and Université de Montréal.

CONFLICT OF INTEREST

The author(s) confirm that this chapter content has no conflict of interest.

REFERENCES

[1]   Molitch ME, Steffes MW, Cleary PA, Nathan DM. Baseline analysis of renal function in the Diabetes Control and Complications Trial. The Diabetes Control and Complications Trial Research Group. Kidney Int 1993; 43(3): 668-74.

[2]   Dahl-Jorgensen K, Bjoro T, Kierulf P, Sandvik L, Bangstad HJ, Hanssen KF. Long-term glycemic control and kidney function in insulin-dependent diabetes mellitus. Kidney Int 1992; 41(4): 920-3.

[3]   The effect of intensive treatment of diabetes on the development and progression of long-term complications in insulin-dependent diabetes mellitus. The Diabetes Control and Complications Trial Research Group. N Engl J Med 1993; 30;329(14): 977-86.

[4]   Nathan DM, Cleary PA, Backlund JY, *et al*. Intensive diabetes treatment and cardiovascular disease in patients with type 1 diabetes. N Engl J Med 2005; 22;353(25): 2643-53.

[5]   Vardanyan M, Parkin E, Gruessner C, Rodriguez Rilo HL. Pancreas *vs.* islet transplantation: a call on the future. Curr Opin Organ Transplant 2009; 15(1): 124-30.

[6]   Ballinger WF, Lacy PE. Transplantation of intact pancreatic islets in rats. Surgery 1972; 72(2): 175-86.

[7]   Tzakis AG, Ricordi C, Alejandro R, *et al*. Pancreatic islet transplantation after upper abdominal exenteration and liver replacement. Lancet 1990; 336(8712): 402-5.

[8]   Brendel M HB, Schulz A, Bretzel R. International Islet Transplant Registry Report. Newsletter2001.

[9]   Shapiro AM, Lakey JR, Ryan EA, *et al*. Islet transplantation in seven patients with type 1 diabetes mellitus using a glucocorticoid-free immunosuppressive regimen. N Engl J Med 2000; 343(4): 230-8.

[10]   Koh A SP, James Shapiro AM. Clinical Trials of Islet Transplantation - Experience of the Edmonton Group and the International Multicenter Trial. In: Hallé J.P. dVP, Rosenberg L., editor. The Bioartificial Pancreas and other Biohybrid Therapies: Research Signpost 2009. p. 403-24.

[11]   Ryan EA, Paty BW, Senior PA, *et al*. Five-year follow-up after clinical islet transplantation. Diabetes 2005; 54(7): 2060-9.

[12]   Ryan EA, Lakey JR, Rajotte RV, *et al*. Clinical outcomes and insulin secretion after islet transplantation with the Edmonton protocol. Diabetes 2001; 50(4): 710-9.

[13]   Senior PA, Zeman M, Paty BW, *et al*. Changes in renal function after clinical islet transplantation: four-year observational study. Am J Transplant 2007; 7(1): 91-8.

[14]   Ritz-Laser B, Oberholzer J, Toso C, Brulhart MC, Zakrzewska K, Ris F, *et al*. Molecular detection of circulating beta-cells after islet transplantation. Diabetes 2002; 51(3): 557-61.

[15]   Barshes NR, Wyllie S, Goss JA. Inflammation-mediated dysfunction and apoptosis in pancreatic islet transplantation: implications for intrahepatic grafts. J Leukoc Biol 2005; 77(5): 587-97.

[16]   Alejandro R, Cutfield RG, Shienvold FL, *et al*. Natural history of intrahepatic canine islet cell autografts. J Clin Invest 1986; 78(5): 1339-48.

[17]   Davalli AM, Ogawa Y, Ricordi C, *et al.* A selective decrease in the beta cell mass of human islets transplanted into diabetic nude mice. Transplantation 1995 27; 59(6): 817-20.

[18]   Bertuzzi F, Ricordi C. Prediction of clinical outcome in islet allotransplantation. Diabetes Care 2007; 30(2): 410-7.

[19]   Bottino R, Fernandez LA, Ricordi C, *et al.* Transplantation of allogeneic islets of Langerhans in the rat liver: effects of macrophage depletion on graft survival and microenvironment activation. Diabetes 1998; 47(3): 316-23.

[20]   Pileggi A, Ribeiro MM, Hogan AR, *et al.* Effects of pancreas cold ischemia on islet function and quality. Transplant Proc 2009; 41(5): 1808-9.

[21]   Wang RN, Rosenberg L. Maintenance of beta-cell function and survival following islet isolation requires re-establishment of the islet-matrix relationship. J Endocrinol 1999; 163(2): 181-90.

[22]   Rosenberg L, Wang R, Paraskevas S, Maysinger D. Structural and functional changes resulting from islet isolation lead to islet cell death. Surgery 1999; 126(2): 393-8.

[23]   Paraskevas S, Duguid WP, Maysinger D, Feldman L, Agapitos D, Rosenberg L. Apoptosis occurs in freshly isolated human islets under standard culture conditions. Transplant Proc 1997; 29(1-2): 750-2.

[24]   Ilieva A, Yuan S, Wang RN, Agapitos D, Hill DJ, Rosenberg L. Pancreatic islet cell survival following islet isolation: the role of cellular interactions in the pancreas. J Endocrinol 1999; 161(3): 357-64.

[25]   Lim F, Sun AM. Microencapsulated islets as bioartificial endocrine pancreas. Science 1980; 210(4472): 908-10.

[26]   Soon-Shiong P, Feldman E, Nelson R, *et al.* Successful reversal of spontaneous diabetes in dogs by intraperitoneal microencapsulated islets. Transplantation 1992; 54(5): 769-74.

[27]   Hasse C, Klock G, Schlosser A, Zimmermann U, Rothmund M. Parathyroid allotransplantation without immunosuppression. Lancet 1997; 350(9087): 1296-7.

[28]   Soon-Shiong P, Heintz RE, Merideth N, *et al.* Insulin independence in a type 1 diabetic patient after encapsulated islet transplantation. Lancet 1994; 343(8903): 950-1.

[29]   Calafiore R, Basta G, Luca G, *et al.* Microencapsulated pancreatic islet allografts into nonimmunosuppressed patients with type 1 diabetes: first two cases. Diabetes Care 2006; 29(1): 137-8.

[30]   Iwata H, Amemiya H, Matsuda T, Takano H, Hayashi R, Akutsu T. Evaluation of microencapsulated islets in agarose gel as bioartificial pancreas by studies of hormone secretion in culture and by xenotransplantation. Diabetes 1989; 38 Suppl 1: 224-5.

[31]   Dautzenberg H, Schuldt U, Grasnick G, *et al.* Development of cellulose sulfate-based polyelectrolyte complex microcapsules for medical applications. Annals of the New York Acad of Sci1999; 875: 46-63.

[32]   Lohr M, Muller P, Karle P, Stange J, Mitzner S, Jesnowski R, *et al.* Targeted chemotherapy by intratumour injection of encapsulated cells engineered to produce CYP2B1, an ifosfamide activating cytochrome P450. Gene Ther 1998; 5(8): 1070-8.

[33]   Zielinski BA, Aebischer P. Chitosan as a matrix for mammalian cell encapsulation. Biomaterials 1994; 15(13): 1049-56.

[34]   Dawson RM, Broughton RL, Stevenson WT, Sefton MV. Microencapsulation of CHO cells in a hydroxyethyl methacrylate-methyl methacrylate copolymer. Biomaterials 1987; 8(5): 360-6.

[35] Kessler L, Pinget M, Aprahamian M, Dejardin P, Damge C. *In vitro* and *in vivo* studies of the properties of an artificial membrane for pancreatic islet encapsulation. Horm Metab Res 1991; 23(7): 312-7.

[36] Cruise GM, Hegre OD, Lamberti FV, *et al*. *In vitro* and *in vivo* performance of porcine islets encapsulated in interfacially photopolymerized poly(ethylene glycol) diacrylate membranes. Cell Trans 1999; 8(3): 293-306.

[37] Fritschy WM, Wolters GH, van Schilfgaarde R. Effect of alginate-polylysine-alginate microencapsulation on *in vitro* insulin release from rat pancreatic islets. Diabetes 1991; 40(1): 37-43.

[38] Remminghorst U, Rehm BH. Bacterial alginates: from biosynthesis to applications. Biotechnol Lett 2006; 28(21): 1701-12.

[39] Hommel M SA, Goosen MFA, inventor. Canada 1984.

[40] Halle JP, Leblond FA, Pariseau JF, Jutras P, Brabant MJ, Lepage Y. Studies on small (< 300 microns) microcapsules: II--Parameters governing the production of alginate beads by high voltage electrostatic pulses. Cell Transplant 1994; 3(5): 365-72.

[41] Lum ZP, Krestow M, Tai IT, Vacek I, Sun AM. Xenografts of rat islets into diabetic mice. An evaluation of new smaller capsules. Transplantation 1992; 53(6): 1180-3.

[42] De Vos P, De Haan B, Pater J, Van Schilfgaarde R. Association between capsule diameter, adequacy of encapsulation, and survival of microencapsulated rat islet allografts. Transplantation 1996; 62(7): 893-9.

[43] King A, Sandler S, Andersson A. The effect of host factors and capsule composition on the cellular overgrowth on implanted alginate capsules. J Biomed Mater Res 2001; 57(3): 374-83.

[44] Strand BL, Ryan TL, In't Veld P, *et al*. Poly-L-Lysine induces fibrosis on alginate microcapsules *via* the induction of cytokines. Cell Transplant 2001; 10(3): 263-75.

[45] Haug A, Smidsrød, Olav. Selectivity of Some Anionic Polymers for Divalent Metal Ions. Acta Chem Scand 1970; 24: 843-54.

[46] Ricordi C, Gray DW, Hering BJ, *et al*. Islet isolation assessment in man and large animals. Acta Diabetol Lat 1990; 27(3): 185-95.

[47] Morini S, Braun M, Onori P, *et al*. Morphological changes of isolated rat pancreatic i slets: a structural, ultrastructural and morphometric study. J Anat 2006; 209(3): 381-92.

[48] Brissova M, Fowler MJ, Nicholson WE, *et al*. Assessment of human pancreatic islet architecture and composition by laser scanning confocal microscopy. J Histochem Cytochem 2005; 53(9): 1087-97.

[49] Orci L, Unger RH. Functional subdivision of islets of Langerhans and possible role of D cells. Lancet 1975; 2(7947): 1243-4.

[50] Cabrera O, Berman DM, Kenyon NS, Ricordi C, Berggren PO, Caicedo A. The unique cytoarchitecture of human pancreatic islets has implications for islet cell function. Proc Natl Acad Sci U S A 2006; 103(7): 2334-9.

[51] Eberhard D, Lammert E. The pancreatic beta-cell in the islet and organ community. Curr Opin Genet Dev 2009; 19(5): 469-75.

[52] Hopcroft DW, Mason DR, Scott RS. Structure-function relationships in pancreatic islets: support for intraislet modulation of insulin secretion. Endocrinology 1985; 117(5): 2073-80.

[53] Bosco D, Orci L, Meda P. Homologous but not heterologous contact increases the insulin secretion of individual pancreatic B-cells. Exp Cell Res 1989; 184(1): 72-80.

[54]   Hauge-Evans AC, Squires PE, Persaud SJ, Jones PM. Pancreatic beta-cell-to-beta-cell interactions are required for integrated responses to nutrient stimuli: enhanced Ca2+ and insulin secretory responses of MIN6 pseudoislets. Diabetes 1999; 48(7): 1402-8.

[55]   Serre-Beinier V, Bosco D, Zulianello L, *et al.* Cx36 makes channels coupling human pancreatic beta-cells, and correlates with insulin expression. Hum Mol Genet 2009; 18(3): 428-39.

[56]   Cirulli V, Baetens D, Rutishauser U, Halban PA, Orci L, Rouiller DG. Expression of neural cell adhesion molecule (N-CAM) in rat islets and its role in islet cell type segregation. J Cell Sci 1994; 107 (Pt 6): 1429-36.

[57]   Rouiller DG, Cirulli V, Halban PA. Uvomorulin mediates calcium-dependent aggregation of islet cells, whereas calcium-independent cell adhesion molecules distinguish between islet cell types. Dev Biol 1991; 148(1): 233-42.

[58]   Dahl U, Sjodin A, Semb H. Cadherins regulate aggregation of pancreatic beta-cells *in vivo*. Development 1996; 122(9): 2895-902.

[59]   Carvell MJ, Marsh PJ, Persaud SJ, Jones PM. E-cadherin interactions regulate beta-cell proliferation in islet-like structures. Cell Physiol Biochem 2007; 20(5): 617-26.

[60]   Rogers GJ, Hodgkin MN, Squires PE. E-cadherin and cell adhesion: a role in architecture and function in the pancreatic islet. Cell Physiol Biochem 2007; 20(6): 987-94.

[61]   Bosco D, Rouiller DG, Halban PA. Differential expression of E-cadherin at the surface of rat beta-cells as a marker of functional heterogeneity. J Endocrinol 2007; 194(1): 21-9.

[62]   Konstantinova I, Lammert E. Microvascular development: learning from pancreatic islets. Bioessays 2004; 26(10): 1069-75.

[63]   Lifson N, Lassa CV, Dixit PK. Relation between blood flow and morphology in islet organ of rat pancreas. Am J Physiol 1985; 249(1 Pt 1): E43-8.

[64]   Lifson N, Kramlinger KG, Mayrand RR, Lender EJ. Blood flow to the rabbit pancreas with special reference to the islets of Langerhans. Gastroenterology 1980; 79(3): 466-73.

[65]   Jansson L, Hellerstrom C. Stimulation by glucose of the blood flow to the pancreatic islets of the rat. Diabetologia 1983; 25(1): 45-50.

[66]   Brissova M, Shostak A, Shiota M, *et al.* Pancreatic islet production of vascular endothelial growth factor-A is essential for islet vascularization, revascularization, and function. Diabetes 2006; 55(11): 2974-85.

[67]   Berg JM. WH Freeman and cie; 2002.

[68]   Hengartner MO. The biochemistry of apoptosis. Nature 2000; 407(6805): 770-6.

[69]   Boatright KM, Salvesen GS. Mechanisms of caspase activation. Curr Opin Cell Biol. 2003; 15(6): 725-31.

[70]   Emamaullee JA, Shapiro AM. Interventional strategies to prevent beta-cell apoptosis in islet transplantation. Diabetes 2006; 55(7): 1907-14.

[71]   Wang GL, Jiang BH, Rue EA, Semenza GL. Hypoxia-inducible factor 1 is a basic-helix-loop-helix-PAS heterodimer regulated by cellular O2 tension. Proc Natl Acad Sci U S A 1995; 92(12): 5510-4.

[72]   Ivan M, Haberberger T, Gervasi DC, *et al.* Biochemical purification and pharmacological inhibition of a mammalian prolyl hydroxylase acting on hypoxia-inducible factor. Proc Natl Acad Sci U S A 2002; 99(21): 13459-64.

[73]   Kallio PJ, Wilson WJ, O'Brien S, Makino Y, Poellinger L. Regulation of the hypoxia-inducible transcription factor 1alpha by the ubiquitin-proteasome pathway. J Biol Chem 1999; 274(10): 6519-25.

[74] Weidemann A, Johnson RS. Biology of HIF-1alpha. Cell Death Differ 2008; 15(4): 621-7.

[75] Patel SA, Simon MC. Biology of hypoxia-inducible factor-2alpha in development and disease. Cell Death Differ 2008; (4): 628-34.

[76] Brusselmans K, Bono F, Maxwell P, *et al.* Hypoxia-inducible factor-2alpha (HIF-2alpha) is involved in the apoptotic response to hypoglycemia but not to hypoxia. J Biol Chem 2001; 276(42): 39192-6.

[77] Maynard MA, Evans AJ, Shi W, Kim WY, Liu FF, Ohh M. Dominant-negative HIF-3 alpha 4 suppresses VHL-null renal cell carcinoma progression. Cell Cycle 2007; 6(22): 2810-6.

[78] Dong Z, Venkatachalam MA, Wang J, *et al.* Up-regulation of apoptosis inhibitory protein IAP-2 by hypoxia. Hif-1-independent mechanisms. J Biol Chem 2001; 276(22): 18702-9.

[79] Bruick RK. Expression of the gene encoding the proapoptotic Nip3 protein is induced by hypoxia. Proc Natl Acad Sci U S A 2000; 97(16): 9082-7.

[80] Carmeliet P, Dor Y, Herbert JM, *et al.* Role of HIF-1alpha in hypoxia-mediated apoptosis, cell proliferation and tumour angiogenesis. Nature 1998; 394(6692): 485-90.

[81] Dionne KE, Colton CK, Yarmush ML. Effect of hypoxia on insulin secretion by isolated rat and canine islets of Langerhans. Diabetes 1993; 42(1): 12-21.

[82] de Groot M, Schuurs TA, Keizer PP, Fekken S, Leuvenink HG, van Schilfgaarde R. Response of encapsulated rat pancreatic islets to hypoxia. Cell Transplant 2003; 12(8): 867-75.

[83] Miao G, Ostrowski RP, Mace J, *et al.* Dynamic production of hypoxia-inducible factor-1alpha in early transplanted islets. Am J Transplant 2006; 6(11): 2636-43.

[84] Greijer AE, van der Wall E. The role of hypoxia inducible factor 1 (HIF-1) in hypoxia induced apoptosis. J Clin Pathol 2004; 57(10): 1009-14.

[85] Moritz W, Meier F, Stroka DM, *et al.* Apoptosis in hypoxic human pancreatic islets correlates with HIF-1alpha expression. FASEB J 2002; 16(7): 745-7.

[86] Ryu GR, Lee MK, Lee E, *et al.* Activation of AMP-activated protein kinase mediates acute and severe hypoxic injury to pancreatic beta cells. Biochem Biophys Res Commun 2009; 386(2): 356-62.

[87] Mohseni Salehi Monfared SS, Larijani B, Abdollahi M. Islet transplantation and antioxidant management: a comprehensive review. World J Gastroenterol 2009; 15(10): 1153-61.

[88] Ko SH, Ryu GR, Kim S, *et al.* Inducible nitric oxide synthase-nitric oxide plays an important role in acute and severe hypoxic injury to pancreatic beta cells. Transplantation 2008; 85(3): 323-30.

[89] Brune B, von Knethen A, Sandau KB. Nitric oxide and its role in apoptosis. Eur J Pharmacol 1998; 351(3): 261-72.

[90] Henningsson R, Salehi A, Lundquist I. Role of nitric oxide synthase isoforms in glucose-stimulated insulin release. Am J Physiol Cell Physiol 2002; 283(1): C296-304.

[91] Gu L, Rutledge B, Fiorillo J, *et al. In vivo* properties of monocyte chemoattractant protein-1. J Leukoc Biol 1997; 62(5): 577-80.

[92] Carlsson PO, Palm F, Andersson A, Liss P. Markedly decreased oxygen tension in transplanted rat pancreatic islets irrespective of the implantation site. Diabetes 2001; 50(3): 489-95.

[93] Carlsson PO, Liss P, Andersson A, Jansson L. Measurements of oxygen tension in native and transplanted rat pancreatic islets. Diabetes 1998; 47(7): 1027-32.

[94]   Carlsson PO, Palm F, Andersson A, Liss P. Chronically decreased oxygen tension in rat pancreatic islets transplanted under the kidney capsule. Transplantation 2000; 69(5): 761-6.

[95]   Mattsson G, Jansson L, Carlsson PO. Decreased vascular density in mouse pancreatic islets after transplantation. Diabetes 2002; 51(5): 1362-6.

[96]   Menger MD, Jaeger S, Walter P, Feifel G, Hammersen F, Messmer K. Angiogenesis and hemodynamics of microvasculature of transplanted islets of Langerhans. Diabetes 1989; 38 Suppl 1: 199-201.

[97]   Mendola JF, Goity C, Fernandez-Alvarez J, *et al.* Immunocytochemical study of pancreatic islet revascularization in islet isograft. Effect of hyperglycemia of the recipient and of *in vitro* culture of islets. Transplantation 1994; 57(5): 725-30.

[98]   Lau J, Carlsson PO. Low revascularization of human islets when experimentally transplanted into the liver. Transplantation 2009; 87(3): 322-5.

[99]   Schrezenmeir J, Kirchgessner J, Gero L, Kunz LA, Beyer J, Mueller-Klieser W. Effect of microencapsulation on oxygen distribution in islets organs. Transplantation 1994; 57(9): 1308-14.

[100]   Schrezenmeir J, Gero L, Laue C, *et al.* The role of oxygen supply in islet transplantation. Transplant Proc 1992; 24(6): 2925-9.

[101]   Avgoustiniatos ES, Colton CK. Effect of external oxygen mass transfer resistances on viability of immunoisolated tissue. Ann N Y Acad Sci 1997; 831: 145-67.

[102]   McClelland RE, Coger RN. Use of micropathways to improve oxygen transport in a hepatic system. J Biomech Eng 2000; 122(3): 268-73.

[103]   Folkman J, Hochberg M. Self-regulation of growth in three dimensions. J Exp Med 1973; 138(4): 745-53.

[104]   Klossner J, Kivisaari J, Niinikoski J. Oxygen and carbon dioxide tensions in the abdominal cavity and colonic wall of the rabbit. Am J Surg 1974; 127(6): 711-5.

[105]   Dufrane D, Steenberghe M, Goebbels RM, Saliez A, Guiot Y, Gianello P. The influence of implantation site on the biocompatibility and survival of alginate encapsulated pig islets in rats. Biomaterials 2006; 27(17): 3201-8.

[106]   Langlois G, Dusseault J, Bilodeau S, Tam SK, Magassouba D, Halle JP. Direct effect of alginate purification on the survival of islets immobilized in alginate-based microcapsules. Acta Biomater 2009; 5(9): 3433-40.

[107]   Robitaille R, Dusseault J, Henley N, Rosenberg L, Halle JP. Insulin-like growth factor II allows prolonged blood glucose normalization with a reduced islet cell mass transplantation. Endocrinology 2003; 144(7): 3037-45.

[108]   Dusseault J, Langlois G, Meunier MC, Menard M, Perreault C, Halle JP. The effect of covalent cross-links between the membrane components of microcapsules on the dissemination of encapsulated malignant cells. Biomaterials 2008; 29(7): 917-24.

[109]   Lehmann R, Zuellig RA, Kugelmeier P, *et al.* Superiority of small islets in human islet transplantation. Diabetes 2007; 56(3): 594-603.

[110]   MacGregor RR, Williams SJ, Tong PY, Kover K, Moore WV, Stehno-Bittel L. Small rat islets are superior to large islets in *in vitro* function and in transplantation outcomes. Am J Physiol Endocrinol Metab 2006; 290(5): E771-9.

[111]   Buchwald P. FEM-based oxygen consumption and cell viability models for avascular pancreatic islets. Theor Biol Med Model 2009; 6:5.

[112]   Zhang WJ, Laue C, Hyder A, Schrezenmeir J. Purity of alginate affects the viability and fibrotic overgrowth of encapsulated porcine islet xenografts. Transplant Proc 2001; 33(7-8): 3517-9.

[113]   Skjak-Braek G, Murano E, Paoletti S. Alginate as immobilization material. II: Determination of polyphenol contaminants by fluorescence spectroscopy, and evaluation of methods for their removal. Biotechnol Bioeng 1989; 33(1): 90-4.

[114]   Tam SK, Dusseault J, Polizu S, Menard M, Halle JP, Yahia L. Impact of residual contamination on the biofunctional properties of purified alginates used for cell encapsulation. Biomaterials 2006; 27(8): 1296-305.

[115]   De Vos P, De Haan BJ, Wolters GH, Strubbe JH, Van Schilfgaarde R. Improved biocompatibility but limited graft survival after purification of alginate for microencapsulation of pancreatic islets. Diabetologia 1997; 40(3): 262-70.

[116]   Mallett AG, Korbutt GS. Alginate modification improves long-term survival and function of transplanted encapsulated islets. Tissue Eng Part A 2009; 15(6): 1301-9.

[117]   Klock G, Pfeffermann A, Ryser C, Grohn P, Kuttler B, Hahn HJ, *et al.* Biocompatibility of mannuronic acid-rich alginates. Biomaterials 1997; 18(10): 707-13.

[118]   Zimmermann U, Klock G, Federlin K, *et al.* Production of mitogen-contamination free alginates with variable ratios of mannuronic acid to guluronic acid by free flow electrophoresis. Electrophoresis 1992; 13(5): 269-74.

[119]   Orive G, Ponce S, Hernandez RM, Gascon AR, Igartua M, Pedraz JL. Biocompatibility of microcapsules for cell immobilization elaborated with different type of alginates. Biomaterials 2002; 23(18): 3825-31.

[120]   Menard M, Dusseault J, Langlois G, *et al.* Role of protein contaminants in the immunogenicity of alginates. J Biomed Mater Res B Appl Biomater 2010; 93(2): 333-40.

[121]   Robitaille R, Dusseault J, Henley N, Desbiens K, Labrecque N, Halle JP. Inflammatory response to peritoneal implantation of alginate-poly-L-lysine microcapsules. Biomaterials 2005; 26(19): 4119-27.

[122]   de Vos P, Smedema I, van Goor H, *et al.* Association between macrophage activation and function of micro-encapsulated rat islets. Diabetologia 2003; 46(5): 666-73.

[123]   Cardozo AK, Proost P, Gysemans C, Chen MC, Mathieu C, Eizirik DL. IL-1beta and IFN-gamma induce the expression of diverse chemokines and IL-15 in human and rat pancreatic islet cells, and in islets from pre-diabetic NOD mice. Diabetologia 2003; 46(2): 255-66.

[124]   Kulseng B, Thu B, Espevik T, Skjak-Braek G. Alginate polylysine microcapsules as immune barrier: permeability of cytokines and immunoglobulins over the capsule membrane. Cell Transplant 1997; 6(4): 387-94.

[125]   de Vos P, de Haan BJ, de Haan A, van Zanten J, Faas MM. Factors influencing functional survival of microencapsulated islet grafts. Cell Transplant 2004; 13(5): 515-24.

[126]   De Vos P, Hillebrands JL, De Haan BJ, Strubbe JH, Van Schilfgaarde R. Efficacy of a prevascularized expanded polytetrafluoroethylene solid support system as a transplantation site for pancreatic islets. Transplantation 1997; 63(6): 824-30.

[127]   Petruzzo P, Pibiri L, De Giudici MA, *et al.* Xenotransplantation of microencapsulated pancreatic islets contained in a vascular prosthesis: preliminary results. Transpl Int 1991; 4(4): 200-4.

[128]   Bloch K, Papismedov E, Yavriyants K, Vorobeychik M, Beer S, Vardi P. Photosynthetic oxygen generator for bioartificial pancreas. Tissue Eng 2006; 12(2): 337-44.

[129]   Zimmermann U, Noth U, Grohn P, *et al.* Non-invasive evaluation of the location, the functional integrity and the oxygen supply of implants: 19F nuclear magnetic resonance imaging of perfluorocarbon-loaded Ba2+-alginate beads. Artif Cells Blood Substit Immobil Biotechnol 2000; 28(2): 129-46.

[130] Maillard E, Sanchez-Dominguez M, Kleiss C, *et al*. Perfluorocarbons: new tool for islets preservation *in vitro*. Transplant Proc 2008; 40(2): 372-4.

[131] Mendoza V, Klein D, Ichii H, *et al*. Protection of islets in culture by delivery of oxygen binding neuroglobin *via* protein transduction. Transplant Proc 2005 Jan-; 37(1): 237-40.

[132] Tilakaratne HK, Yang B, Hunter SK, Andracki ME, Rodgers VG. Can myoglobin expression in pancreatic beta cells improve insulin secretion under hypoxia? An exploratory study with transgenic porcine islets. Artif Organs 2007; 31(7): 521-31.

[133] Stagner JI, Parthasarathy SN, Wyler K, Parthasarathy RN. Protection from ischemic c ell death by the induction of cytoglobin. Transplant Proc 2005 Oct; 37(8): 3452-3.

[134] Mysore TB, Shinkel TA, Collins J, *et al*. Overexpression of glutathione peroxidase with two isoforms of superoxide dismutase protects mouse islets from oxidative injury and improves islet graft function. Diabetes 2005; 54(7): 2109-16.

[135] Hyder A, Laue C, Schrezenmeir J. Metabolic aspects of neonatal rat islet hypoxia tolerance. Transpl Int 2010;23(1): 80-9.

[136] Emamaullee JA, Shapiro AM, Rajotte RV, Korbutt G, Elliott JF. Neonatal porcine islets exhibit natural resistance to hypoxia-induced apoptosis. Transplantation 2006; 82(7): 945-52.

[137] Wright JR, Jr., Pohajdak B. Cell therapy for diabetes using piscine islet tissue. Cell Transplant 2001; 10(2): 125-43.

[138] Yang H, Morrison CM, Conlon JM, Laybolt K, Wright JR, Jr. Immunocytochemical characterization of the pancreatic islet cells of the Nile Tilapia (Oreochromis niloticus). Gen Comp Endocrinol 1999; 114(1): 47-56.

[139] Emamaullee JA, Rajotte RV, Liston P, *et al*. XIAP overexpression in human islets prevents early posttransplant apoptosis and reduces the islet mass needed to treat diabetes. Diabetes 2005; 54(9): 2541-8.

[140] Plesner A, Liston P, Tan R, Korneluk RG, Verchere CB. The X-linked inhibitor of apoptosis protein enhances survival of murine islet allografts. Diabetes 2005; 54(9): 2533-40.

[141] Wang J, Cao Y, Chen Y, Gardner P, Steiner DF. Pancreatic beta cells lack a low glucose and O2-inducible mitochondrial protein that augments cell survival. Proc Natl Acad Sci U S A 2006; 103(28): 10636-41.

[142] Kugelmeier P, Nett PC, Zullig R, Lehmann R, Weber M, Moritz W. Expression and hypoxic regulation of the endothelin system in endocrine cells of human and rat pancreatic islets. JOP 2008; 9(2): 133-49.

[143] Dong H, Woo SL. Hepatic insulin production for type 1 diabetes. Trends Endocrinol Metab 2001; 12(10): 441-6.

[144] Alam T, Sollinger HW. Glucose-regulated insulin production in hepatocytes. Transplantation 2002; 74(12): 1781-7.

[145] Yasutomi K, Itokawa Y, Asada H, *et al*. Intravascular insulin gene delivery as potential therapeutic intervention in diabetes mellitus. Biochem Biophys Res Commun 2003; 310(3): 897-903.

[146] Chen NK, Sivalingam J, Tan SY, Kon OL. Plasmid-electroporated primary hepatocytes acquire quasi-physiological secretion of human insulin and restore euglycemia in diabetic mice. Gene Ther 2005; 12(8): 655-67.

[147] Olson DE, Paveglio SA, Huey PU, Porter MH, Thule PM. Glucose-responsive hepatic insulin gene therapy of spontaneously diabetic BB/Wor rats. Hum Gene Ther 2003; 14(15): 1401-13.

[148] Samson SL, Chan L. Gene therapy for diabetes: reinventing the islet. Trends Endocrinol Metab 2006; 17(3): 92-100.

[149] Ricordi C, Lacy PE, Finke EH, Olack BJ, Scharp DW. Automated method for isolation of human pancreatic islets. Diabetes 1988; 37(4): 413-20.

Send Orders of Reprints at reprints@benthamscience.net

Human Trials with Microencapsulated Insulin-Producing Cells: Past, Present and Future

Bernard Tuch[1,2,*], **Vijayaganapathy Vaithilingam**[1,2] **and Jayne Foster**[2]

[1]*Biomedical Materials & Devices, Materials Science & Engineering, CSIRO, Sydney, Australia;* [2]*Former Diabetes Transplant Unit, Prince of Wales Hospital & University of New South Wales, Sydney, Australia*

Abstract: Microencapsulation of insulin-producing cells is a promising strategy to deliver a cell therapy for treatment of type 1 diabetes without the need for anti-rejection drugs. In this Chapter, we describe our experience in producing microcapsules made of barium alginate, and their application pre-clinically in diabetic rodents and pigs before moving to the clinic in a first-in-man trial with encapsulated human islets. Whilst the use of the microcapsules was safe in the clinical trial, we have learnt from the trial that it is necessary to modify the microcapsule to reduce pericapsular fibrosis, and strategies are being implemented to achieve this. Moreover, the supply of human islets for the clinic is quite limited, and we are now making pancreatic progenitors from pluripotent human embryonic stem cells as a much more reliable and larger source of surrogate cells for encapsulation and transplantation. [Clinical Trial Registration Number ACTRN12609000192280 (Australian and New Zealand Clinical Trials Registry)].

Keywords: Microcapsules, insulin-dependent diabetes, islets, pericapsular fibrotic overgrowth, embryonic stem cells, barium alginate, porcine islet-like cell clusters, fetal pancreas, transplantation, clinical trial.

1. INTRODUCTION

Cell therapies for insulin-dependent diabetes originally began in the 1967 when islets were isolated from mice [1] and subsequently transplanted into diabetic recipients. Islets were successfully isolated from cadaveric humans over the next two decades, shown to normalize blood glucose levels in diabetic immunodeficient mice, and then grafted into humans. The first person to achieve

Address correspondence to Bernard Tuch: Biomedical Materials & Devices, Materials Science & Engineering, CSIRO, PO Box 52, North Ryde, Sydney, NSW 1670 Australia; Tel: 61 2 9490 5053; Fax: 61 2 9490 5483; E-mail: bernie.tuch@csiro.au

normoglycaemia by this approach was in 1989 with the doyen of islet transplantation Paul Lacy leading the way, ably assisted by David Scharp and Camillo Ricordi [2]. As might be expected, immunosuppression was required to prevent rejection of the allografted tissue.

A decade later, the success rate of islet transplantation was quite low with only 12% of type 1 diabetic recipients remaining off insulin one year after receiving an intraportal injection of islets. In 2000, researchers in Edmonton revolutionised the field by showing that if non-steroidal immunosuppressive therapy was used, 100% of recipients could still be insulin-free at one year [3]. However, with time post transplant, most recipients require re-administration of insulin, with < 20% of recipients still remaining insulin free at six years [4]. In those are the groups with the most experience and are highly selective about which islets to transplant, for example, those in Minneapolis and at the University of Illinois in Chicago, success rates at five years are now 60% (J. Oberholzer, personal communication).

Regardless, those who qualify to receive an islet transplant are limited because of the risks of the anti-rejection drugs. They cause an increased risk of infection as well as neoplasia, and have a number of side effects, including liver dysfunction, bleeding, mouth ulcers and hypercholesterolaemia, which in the extreme require recipients to cease the medication. Because of these risks, recipients are usually limited to those with unrecognized hypoglycaemic events. In these people, the benefit outweighs the risks. The number of such recipients is therefore quite small. Worldwide there are at least 960 people with type 1 diabetes who have been allografted with human islets [4, 5]. The number of people with type 1 diabetes is thought to be 18.3 million [estimate based on 5% of total world diabetes population of 366 million [6].

2. ALTERNATIVE SOURCE OF BETA CELLS

A second limiting factor for successful islet transplantation is the supply of human islets. Donor pancreases from which islets are isolated are scarce, with a maximum of 10-30 donors per million population per annum. Even where multiple organs are harvested from a donor, the pancreas may not be retrieved, usually for technical reasons, meaning that there are even fewer pancreases available to harvest islets from [7]. In addition, when the pancreas is obtained, it is usually used for whole pancreas transplantation, often combined with a kidney for someone with renal failure. Thus, in Australia, with a population of 22 million, the number of cadaveric donors in 2010 was 309, the number of whole pancreases transplanted was 34, and the number of pancreases from which islets were isolated and used clinically was 12 [7]. Yet, the number of Australians with type 1 diabetes is 143,000. This example illustrates the problem of the shortage of donor pancreases faced in all countries for people with type 1 diabetes trying to overcome the need for insulin administration by transplanting human islets.

Alternative sources of exogenous beta cells include pig islets, stem cells, the non-endocrine component of adult pancreases, and fetal human pancreases. Almost all of these sources will require a strategy to overcome the immune system of the diabetic recipient since the donor cells will be recognized as foreign, and be rejected. The major exception to this is when the cells are autologous in nature, for example, mesenchymal stem cells harvested from bone marrow, peripheral or cord blood [8]. A second possible exception is the use of first trimester human fetal pancreas in which the class II histocompatibility antigens are not yet expressed [9].

3. ENCAPSULATION

The search for a means of transplanting cells from another source without having to use anti-rejection therapy began in 1975 [10], with the placement of cells by Buschard inside an immunoprotective device, a Millipore chamber. Almost two decades later, in 1994, the field became excited when Soon Shiong and colleagues reported it possible for a person with insulin-dependent diabetes to cease insulin injections after receiving encapsulated human islets [11]. The microcapsules used were made of alginate high in guluronic acid content, and coated with poly-L-lysine. The recipient was on immunosuppressive therapy and had received a renal transplant previously. However, as of 2011, there are no other reports of sustained insulin independence in diabetic humans receiving encapsulated human islets, although graft function has been achieved by Calafiore [12, 13] and our own group [14].

The possibility of using encapsulated porcine rather than human islets received a major boost in 1996 when Tony Sun in Toronto reported that diabetic monkeys became normoglycaemic when grafted with microencapsulated pig islets [15]. The efforts of his team were in part reproduced by others in 2010, with Dufrane's group in Belgium achieving euglycaemia for 6 months in diabetic monkeys engrafted with sheets of microencapsulated pig islets [16]. Elliott and colleagues have taken microencapsulated neonatal porcine islet-like cell clusters to the clinic with production of porcine insulin in recipients [17] and a decrease in frequency of hypoglycaemic unawareness.

There are three main types of devices used to transplant cells without using immunosuppression: (a) multiple microcapsules, usually made of alginate [18]; (b) a single diffusion chamber, for example, the Theracyte device [19]; and (c) vascularised devices [20]. There are numerous reviews covering these three types [21-23], and in this chapter, we will concentrate on our own experience, utilizing microcapsules made of barium alginate.

3.1. Barium Alginate Microcapsules

Our foray into the field of encapsulation began in 2001-2, when we learnt the technique from Ulrichs and Mayer during their visits from Würzburg, Germany (Stepwise Protocol 1). They reported the ability of pig islets microencapsulated in ultrapure medium viscosity grade (UP MVG) sodium alginate (NovaMatrix/FMC Biopolymer) to normalize blood glucose levels of diabetic immunocompetent (Wistar) rats [24]. The alginate microcapsules were made with an air-driven droplet generator, and solidified for 2 minutes in 20 mM barium chloride to enhance their stability. Barium forms strong cross-links with the monomers that make up the alginate, guluronic and mannuronic acid. The ratio of these two acids in the capsules was 69:31, the higher guluronic acid content making them more rigid and stable, as compared to capsules made with high mannuronic acid content.

The size of the microcapsules made in our Unit at the University of New South Wales/Prince of Wales Hospital were 200 – 700 µm, but more usually 300 – 500 µm, with the size being controlled by the air pressure and flow rate (Fig. **1**). Capsule pore size, as determined by inverse size exclusion chromatography using pullulan standards [25] was ~250 kDa [26]. This excluded IgM and immune cells, but not IgG, which has a molecular weight of 150 kDa, or chemokines and cytokines, which have molecular weights of <50 kDa.

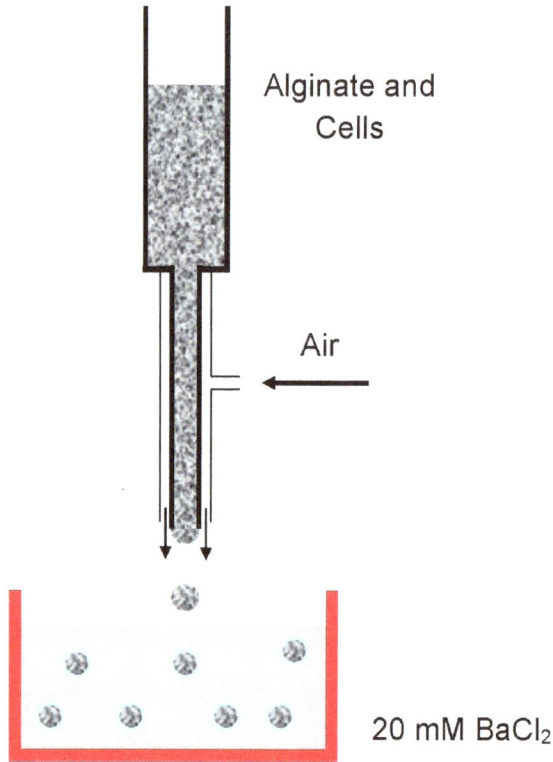

Figure 1: This figure depicts the encapsulation process.

3.2. Encapsulated Human Islets

Human islets placed inside these microcapsules continued to secrete insulin, and the amount increased when beta cell stimuli, especially glucose 20 mM, was added to the culture medium [27]. Insulin content of the islets was unaffected by the encapsulation process, being 222 ± 27 µU/islet when encapsulated and 246 ± 64 µU/islet when non-encapsulated [27]. Importantly, encapsulated human islets infused into the peritoneal cavity of diabetic immunodeficient (NOD/SCID) mice normalized their random blood glucose levels within three days of the surgery [27] and (Stepwise Protocol 2). The blood glucose levels obtained, 4-7 mmol/L, were lower than those found in non-diabetic control mice, 6-10 mmol/L, being akin to the levels found in humans. The fact that islet transplant recipients adopt the blood glucose level of the donor species has been known for some years [28]. Blood glucose levels measured during oral glucose tolerance tests (OGTT) carried out in these normoglycaemic mice were either the same as those of control mice, or lower. Human C-peptide was measurable in mouse plasma, and rose in response to oral glucose administration during the OGTT.

A concern often raised in the field of transplantation is that the number of encapsulated islets required to normalize blood glucose levels in diabetic recipients is greater than the number of non-encapsulated islets to achieve this goal. If this was correct, it would mitigate against this platform technology. We have found that, at least in diabetic immunodeficient mice, 2000 islets is the minimum number needed to achieve euglycaemia, regardless of whether they are encapsulated [27]. The encapsulated islets are placed in the peritoneal cavity, and the non-encapsulated islets beneath the renal capsule. Whilst ideally it would be best if both groups of islets were transplanted at the same site, this is not feasible. Microcapsules are generally too large to be placed beneath the renal capsule of mice, and non-encapsulated islets do not survive well when placed freely in the peritoneal cavity.

A second concern that has been raised in encapsulation studies is that the cells in the core of the microcapsule, may not receive sufficient oxygen and other nutrients to function efficiently. This seems to be an issue especially when encapsulated islets are transplanted subcutaneously [29]. To examine whether encapsulation itself affected the transcriptome of human islets, we organized for microarray analysis to be carried out on encapsulated islets cultured for up to seven days, and compared the data with that from non-encapsulated human islets. Of the thousands of genes present in the islets, only a very small number, 29, were up regulated and 2 down regulated [30]. Analysis of the data using Ingenuity software showed that up-regulated genes were involved mostly in inflammation, especially chemotaxis, and vascularisation. However, protein expression of these genes, as measured by Western Blots, was not altered by encapsulation. That the alteration in gene expression did not translate into altered protein levels raises doubts about the biosignificance of the gene changes. The miRNAs in human islets also were examined and as with the gene analysis, encapsulation had no effect on their expression levels [30]. In summary, encapsulation has no significant adverse effect on overall gene expression. Thus, at least *in vitro*, hypoxia is not an issue, but whether this is so *in vivo* remained to be determined.

To investigate this, encapsulated islets were transplanted into the peritoneal cavity of diabetic mice, where there is a relatively low level of oxygen, after being incubated with desferrioxamine (DFO) 100 μM prior to transplantation. This iron chelator also functions to increase levels of vascular endothelial growth factor, and its downstream agent, hypoxia inducing factor 1-α in human islets [31], thereby conditioning them to hypoxia. With this strategy, the number of islets required to consistently normalize blood glucose levels in diabetic immunodeficient mice was reduced from 2000 to 1000 [31]. When 750 DFO preconditioned islets were grafted into the diabetic mice, normoglycaemia was achieved in 50% of recipients, whereas this was achieved in only 10% of mice receiving unconditioned islets [31]. It is concluded that hypoxia is an issue limiting functional outcomes *in vivo*, at least when the peritoneal cavity was the site of implantation.

4. PREVENTING ALLOGRAFT REJECTION IN ANIMALS

4.1. Mice

Whilst it was helpful to know that our encapsulated human islets would normalize blood glucose levels in diabetic recipient NOD/SCID mice, how they would survive in an allograft situation was unknown. To investigate this, we encapsulated mouse insulin-producing cells (MIN6 cell line) and transplanted these into streptozotocin-induced diabetic immunocompetent BALB/c mice, which have a major difference in the major histocompatibility complex to the MIN6 cells. Animals transplanted with 1×10^7 cells became normoglycaemic within the first three days of being transplanted and remained so until the experiment was terminated at six weeks (Fig. **2a**) [32]. Those receiving $4 - 6 \times 10^6$ cells also became normoglycaemic within 3 days, but then blood glucose levels rose, only to return to normal levels at 7 weeks, and remain normal until the end of the experiment at 10 weeks (Fig. **2b** & **2c**). Mice receiving 2×10^6 cells became normoglycaemic only at six weeks (Fig. **2d**). These data are interpreted to mean that death of some of the encapsulated MIN6 cells occurs shortly after they are transplanted, with dumping of insulin, but the residual cells compensate over the next six weeks, perhaps by proliferation. Confirmation of this hypothesis will require analysis of the encapsulated cells at different times after transplantation, using markers for cell death and proliferation.

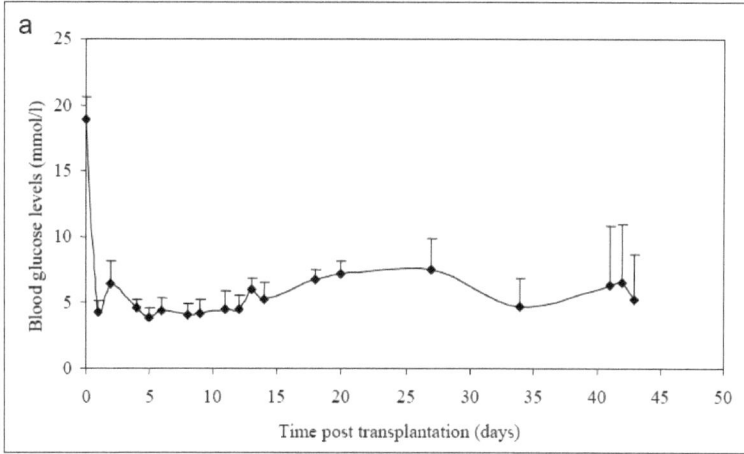

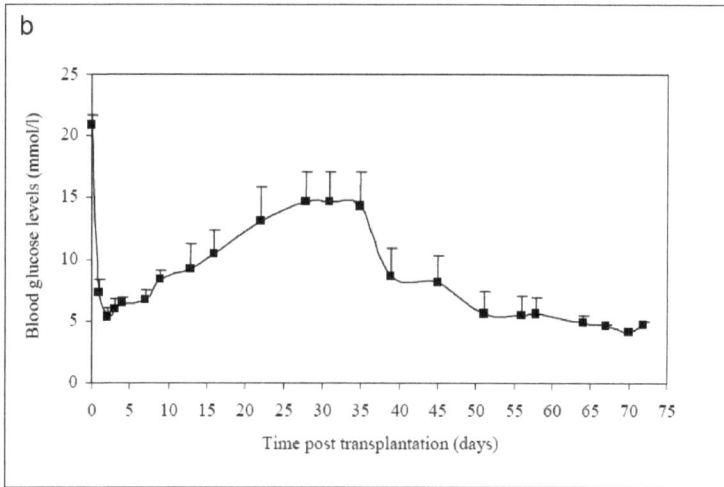

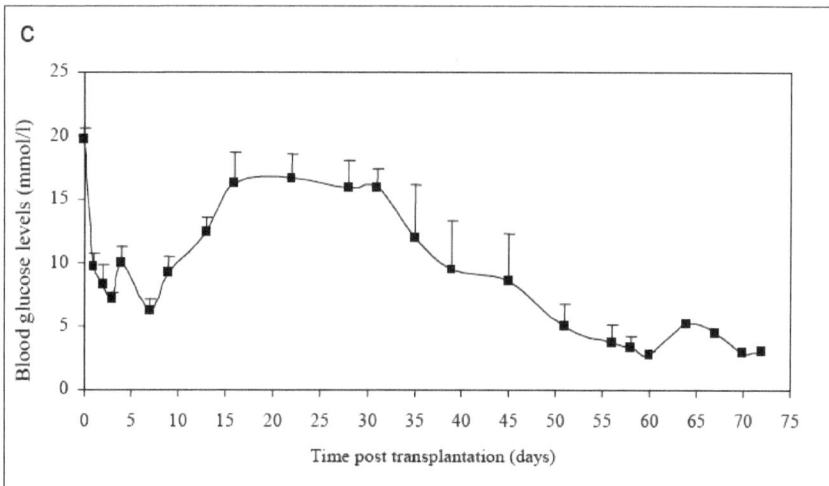

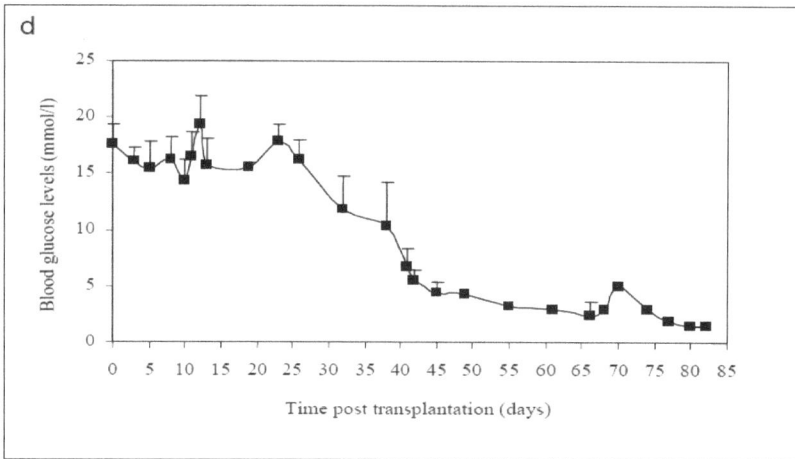

Figure 2: Blood glucose levels of streptozotocin-induced diabetic immunocompetent BALB/c mice transplanted with a) 10×10^6; b) 6×10^6; c) 4×10^6 and d) 2×10^6 encapsulated MIN6 cells (n = 3-6).

Hypoglycaemia was not experienced in mice transplanted with $\leq 1 \times 10^7$ MIN6, perhaps because the cell line was shown to be glucose responsive *in vitro* [32]. However, when greater than this number of cells were grafted, hypoglycaemia occurred, and the mice were euthanized. The microcapsules retrieved from the mice in which normoglycaemia was achieved were clear of fibrosis, and the encapsulated MIN6 cells were viable, as shown by staining mostly for the fluorescent dye, carboxyfluorescein diacetate (CFDA), but not propidium iodide (PI), which stains dead cells [32]. Altering the size of the microcapsules made no significant difference to the time required for 2×10^6 cells to normalize blood glucose levels in recipient diabetic mice. The times post transplantation to achieve normoglycaemia were 31 ± 4, 30 ± 5 and 20 ± 8 days (mean $\pm$ SEM, n = 6) for capsules of diameter 200 - 400, 500 - 700 and 700 – 1000 μm respectively [32].

4.2. Pigs

Next, we addressed the question of whether the results we had obtained in the mice could be achieved in a large animal, the pig. Previously, we had shown that blood glucose levels could be lowered towards normal in diabetic pigs in which non-encapsulated fetal pig islet-like cell clusters (ICCs) were grafted into the thymus gland [33]. Accordingly, we chose to determine if encapsulated fetal porcine ICCs would normalize blood glucose levels of diabetic pigs.

Before carrying out these experiments, we confirmed that encapsulated fetal porcine ICCs were viable, and were able to secrete insulin when exposed to insulinogenic stimuli, such as 10 mM cyclic AMP, 10 mM theophylline, and 20 mM KCl [34]. That these ICCs did not secrete insulin when exposed to glucose 20 mM glucose [34] was expected, as immature beta cells of all species lack this ability [35]. We also showed that these encapsulated immature cells secreted porcine insulin when transplanted into NOD/SCID mice, a process that took between 13 and 68 days, with 10,000 ICCs as the minimal number required to achieve normoglycaemia consistently. The diameter of the microcapsules was a factor examined, with results showing that encapsulated ICCs functioned as efficiently in capsules of diameter 310 μm, as in those three times the diameter [34]. That the ICCs at the centre of the larger capsules did not show necrosis might be explained by the immaturity of the cells, and the ability of immature tissue, as compared to mature islets, to survive under hypoxic conditions.

The pigs we transplanted fetal porcine ICCs into were either Large White Landrace (n = 5) or minipigs (n = 4), of weight 15-20 kg [32]. All animals were normoglycaemic at the time they received ICCs, which had been harvested from the pancreases of one or two litters of fetal pigs aged 75-90 days gestation. The total number of ICCs implanted was 122,000 – 220,000 (average 194,400). Since the average diameter of an ICC was 90 μm, as compared to 150 μm for an adult human islet, this meant that the number of islet equivalents transplanted was only 20,740 – 37,400 (mean 33,060). The ICCs were implanted either in the peritoneal cavity or in an omental pouch with the sac tied off with a purse string non-resorbable suture to assist in identifying it at post mortem (Fig. **3**). Diabetes was induced in recipient pigs usually six days after transplantation, by intravenous injection of 150 mg/kg streptozotocin. The timing of the injection was for reasons of practicality (intravenous access), especially since fetal pig beta cells are resistant to the toxic effects of streptozotocin [36].

Blood glucose levels did decline in the Large White Landrace pigs from a peak of 22 mmol/L to levels of 11 mmol/L at weeks 13-15, but then rose again as the daily dose of insulin being administered, 0.4-0.5 U/kg, was lowered (Fig. **4**). Data were similar regardless of the site of implantation of the ICCs [32]. Glucagon and arginine challenge tests were carried out periodically to ascertain the degree of endogenous beta cell activity. Best results were obtained in the Large White Landrace pigs receiving ICCs in the omental pouch. Two weeks after transplantation, no porcine C-peptide was detected in these animals, but it was at 6 weeks, rising to a peak (73% of the non-diabetic area under the curve) at 14 weeks in the glucagon challenge (Fig. **5**). With the arginine challenge, C-peptide levels became 95% of the non-diabetic area under the curve at 10-18 weeks (Fig. **6**).

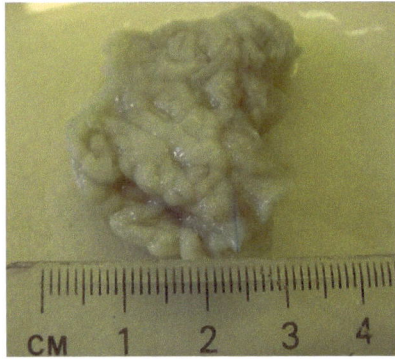

Figure 3: Omental pouch retrieved from diabetic Large White Landrace pig transplanted with encapsulated fetal pig ICCs at 130 days post transplantation.

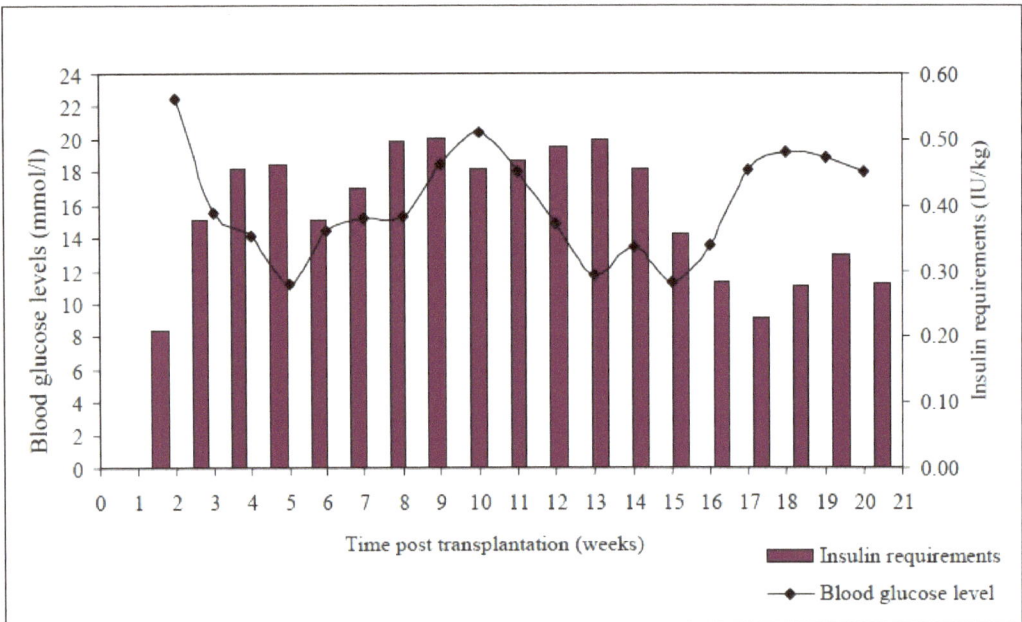

Figure 4: Blood glucose levels and insulin requirements per kilogram bodyweight of Large White Landrace pigs transplanted with encapsulated fetal pig ICCs within an omental pouch (n = 2).

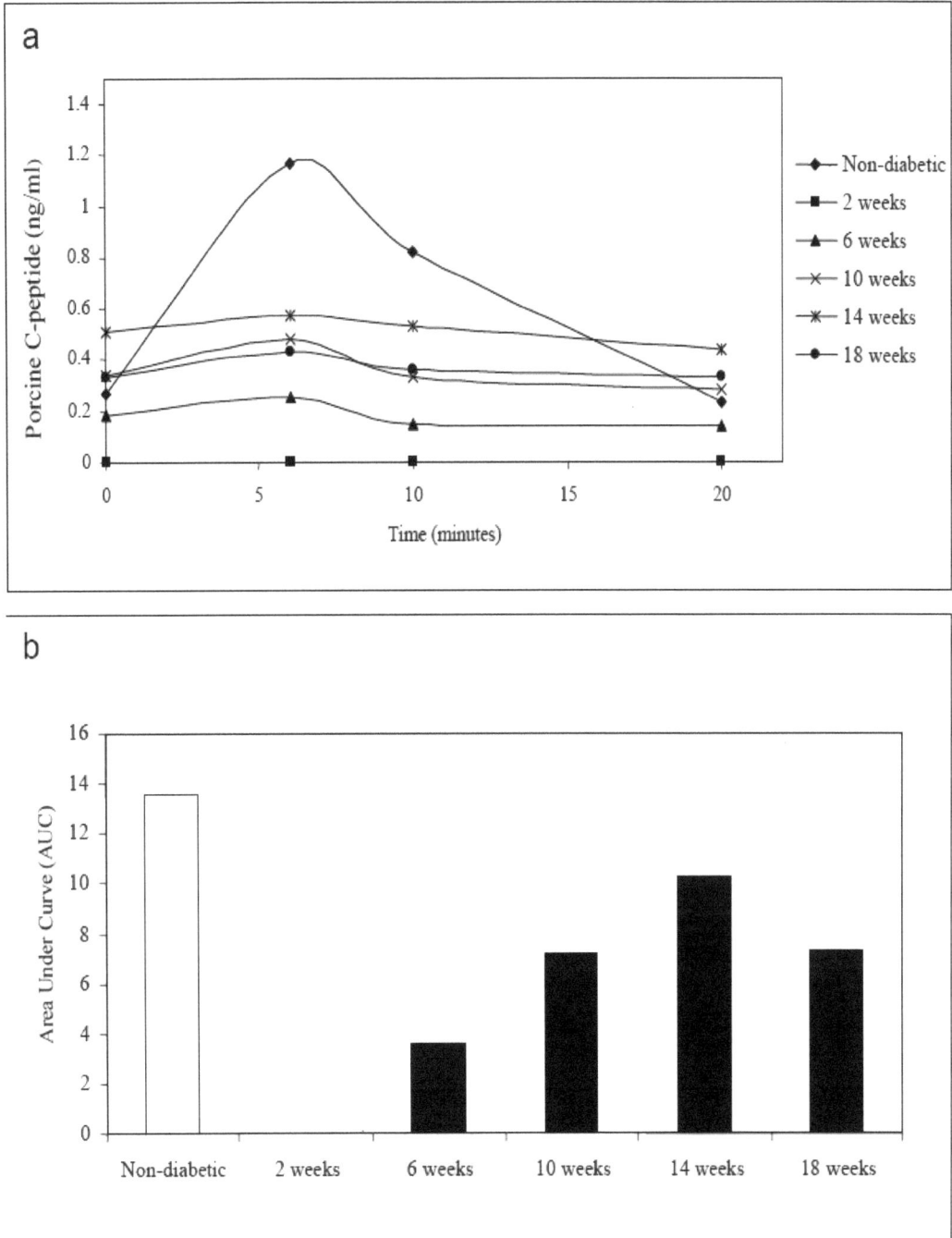

Figure 5: a) Glucagon challenge tests and b) corresponding area under curve analysis performed in Large White Landrace pigs transplanted within an omental pouch prior to induction of diabetes and 2-18 weeks post transplantation (n = 2).

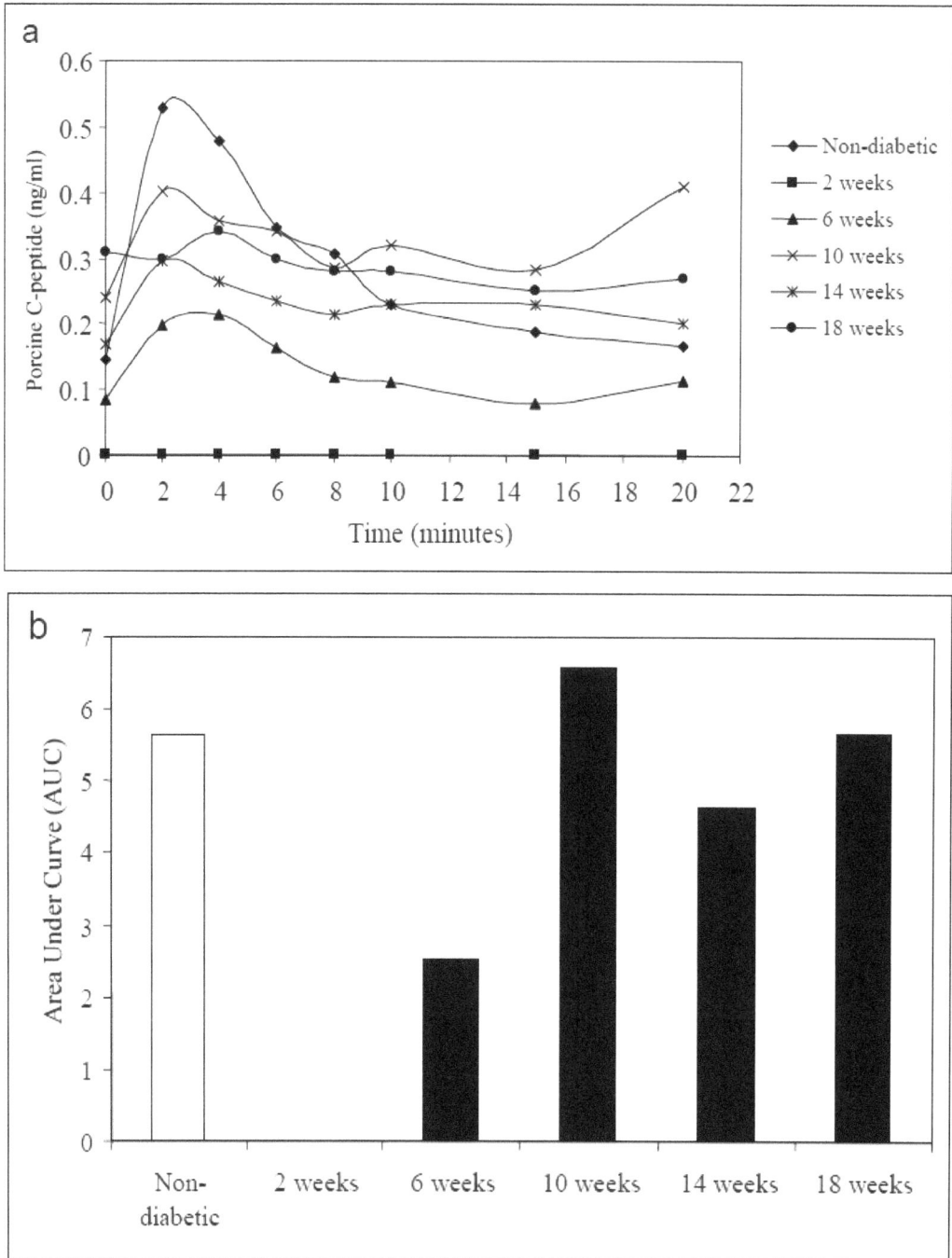

Figure 6: a) Arginine challenge tests and b) corresponding area under curve analysis performed in Large White Landrace pigs transplanted within an omental pouch prior to induction of diabetes and 2-18 weeks post transplantation (n = 2).

Recovery of ICCs from the pigs proved difficult because of the large size of the animals, 90-100 kg for the Large White Landrace pigs and 45-50 kg for the minipigs [32]. ICCs could not be detected within the peritoneum of these animals but they could in the omental pouch in at least one transplanted Large White Landrace pig. Microcapsules here were free of fibrosis and the cells inside appeared intact, as they also did prior to transplantation (Fig. **7**). It would seem that most of the porcine C-peptide in the blood of diabetic pigs was coming from the grafts rather than the residual beta cells in the pig pancreas, the number of insulin-positive cells in an islet being 3 ± 2, c.f., 54 ± 8 for the non-diabetic pigs.

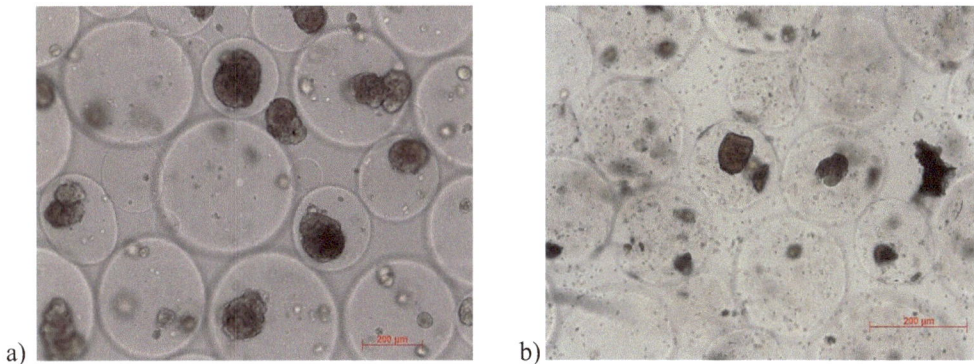

Figure 7: Encapsulated fetal pig ICCs, a) prior to transplantation and b) recovered from the omental pouch of a Large White Landrace pig at 130 days post transplantation.

5. FIRST-IN-MAN HUMAN TRIAL

With the rodent and porcine data all looking promising, a decision was reached to proceed with a first-in-man human trial using encapsulated human islets isolated from cadaveric donors [14]. A total of 14 type 1 diabetic patients were screened and seven enrolled into the trial. Of these, 4 received islets isolated from 8 cadaveric pancreases over a period of 19 months, commencing in February 2006. One person received four preparations, another two, and the others 1 each. Duration of diabetes was 24 – 40 years, and age 38 – 51 years. Those receiving islets were aged 38 -51, weighed < 70 kg, had a body mass index of < 25, and had no endogenous production of C-peptide, as assessed during an arginine stimulation test and in a 24 hour sample of urine. The titre of autoimmune antibodies (ICA512 and glutamic acid decarboxylase) was negative, and renal function was normal.

The protocol used in this study and the details of the encapsulated islets used are described at the end of the chapter.

5.1. Source of Tissue

Adult human pancreases were obtained from deceased donors after informed consent obtained from the next-of-kin by the organ donor co-ordinators of the NSW Red Cross. The criteria for accepting a donor were those adopted by the Islet Core Isolation and Transplant Centre, Justus-Liebig University Giessen, Giessen, Germany. They were:

- age 18-65y.

- body mass index >25.

- duration in intensive care <7 days.

- circulation: no hypotensive periods leading to functional organ damage (rise in serum creatinine or liver transaminases >50%).

- blood glucose level <16.7 mM.

- normal serum amylase & lipase.

- patient history: no evidence of alcohol abuse or chronic pancreatitis.

- absence of infection serologically for HIV 1 & 2, hepatitis B & C, and HTLV 1 & 2.

5.2. Preparation of Islets

The pancreas was removed from the donor and digested to produce islets by intraductal injection of the enzymes collagenase NB1 premium grade and neutral protease NB (Serva, Germany), and gentle mechanical dissociation in a Ricordi chamber. Once the pancreas had been digested, the islets were purified using Ficoll gradient density centrifugation in a refrigerated Cobe 2991 Cell Processor.

Immediately after islet purification, the islets were resuspended in CMRL1066 media containing 5% human albumin, 1% insulin, transferrin and selenium (ITS) and the antibiotics benzyl penicillin (100 µg/ml) and gentamicin (40 µg/ml), and cultured for two to three days before being encapsulated.

5.3. Encapsulation of Islets

On day two to three post-isolation, the islets were taken out of culture and washed with Hanks Balanced Salt Solution then resuspended in 2.2% sodium alginate UP MVG (NovaMatrix/FMC Biopolymer) in a ratio of 1:8. The alginate had a high guluronic acid: mannuronic acid composition, was of GMP grade and sterile. This suspension was transferred to an air-driven droplet generator. Microcapsules of islets and alginate were generated and incubated in a bath of 20 mM barium chloride for two minutes. Supernatant from the settled microcapsules was discarded and the microcapsules washed three times in Hanks Balanced Salt Solution to remove the excess barium. Microcapsules containing the islets, one to two per microcapsule, were placed in CMRL 1066 media containing human albumin, ITS and antibiotics.

5.4. Characterization of Encapsulated Islets

The encapsulated islets were characterized in the following manner:

- Number of islets. Duplicate aliquots (200 µl) of islet suspension were taken after purification, dithizone (stains zinc molecules attached to (pro)insulin in the secretory granules of beta cells) added to the cell suspension and following 5 minutes incubation, islet size and number of islet equivalents estimated. The median number of islet equivalents from the eight islet preparations was 178,200 (range 98,200 – 227,900).

- Diameter of capsules. Duplicate aliquots (200 µl) of the capsule suspension were taken following encapsulation and the diameter of the microcapsules determined. Median average diameter of the eight islet preparations was 340 µm (range 255 – 750).

- Purity. The ratio of islets to exocrine tissue was ascertained after dithizone staining. Median was 68% (range 50 -88).

- Viability. This was assessed with the fluorescent dyes CFDA and PI, and the percentage of viable cells calculated. Median was 73% (range 60 – 80).

- Insulin content. Insulin was extracted from 50 islets (in triplicate), using acid ethanol, and levels of the hormone measured by radioimmunoassay. Median was 1.1 mU/islet equivalent (range 0.1 – 35).

- Insulin secretion. Fifty islets (in triplicate) were exposed to 20 mM glucose for one hour, and the levels of insulin secreted compared to those from islets exposed to 2.8 mM glucose. Median stimulation index was 1.22 (range 1.0 – 2.4).

- Microbial contamination. Prior to transplantation, a sample of culture medium conditioned by the encapsulated islets was collected and added to blood agar, looking for aerobic bacterial organisms. Microorganisms were never detected.

5.5. Transplantation of Encapsulated Islets

Following overnight culture, the encapsulated islets were transferred to transplant media (phenol red-free Hanks Balanced Salt Solution with 5% human albumin), and then injected into the peritoneal cavity of recipients by an experienced radiologist. This required an injection of local anaesthetic to the skin of the periumbilical region and insertion of a plastic 14 g cannula into the peritoneum. Water soluble, non-ionic low osmolar radio-opaque dye was injected through the cannula, and the abdomen visualized fluoroscopically. Only when it had been determined that the cannula was not in the bowel were the encapsulated islets injected. After this, 50 mL transplant media was infused through the catheter to ensure that all microcapsules had entered the peritoneal cavity.

5.6. Medication

Whilst the recipients received no anti-rejection drugs, they did receive the mild anti-inflammatory (and lipid lowering) agent atorvastatin 20 mg, as well as the antioxidants vitamin A 50,000 units, vitamin B6 100 mg and vitamin E 750 units daily. In one recipient, the incretin exenatide 5-10 µg was administered subcutaneously.

5.7. Outcome

All recipients showed evidence of graft function in the immediate post-transplant period (Fig. **8**) and this impacted glycaemic control, with low blood glucose levels experienced requiring a transient reduction in exogenous insulin administration [11]. However, after the end of the first week, the encapsulated islets made no further clinical impact. In one patient, who had received four islet preparations, a low level of urinary (0.06 – 0.34 nmol/L) but not plasma C-peptide was detected for up to 2.5 years after the third infusion.

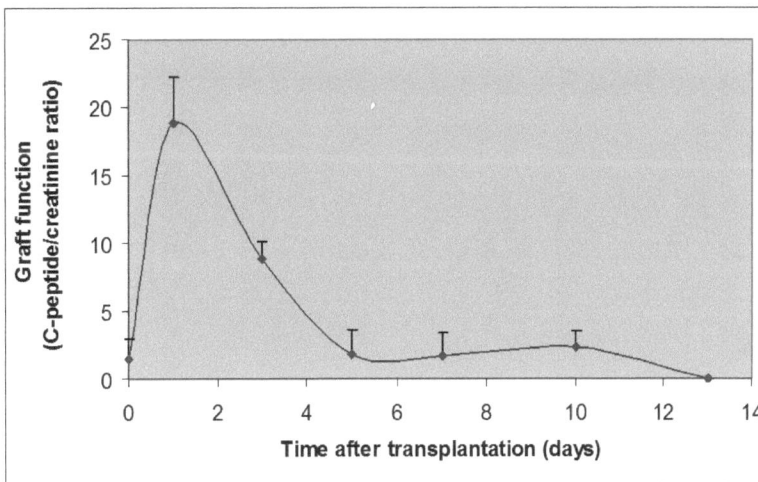

Figure 8: Evidence of transient early graft function of the 4 people with type 1 diabetes transplanted with encapsulated human islets. Two people were transplanted with islets isolated from one pancreas each, one person with islets from two pancreases, and one with islets from four pancreases.

Examination of the peritoneum of this person 15 months after the first infusion (18 days before the third infusion) revealed the microcapsules clumped together in a large number of sites – parietal peritoneum, kidney, spleen (Fig. **9a**), omentum and liver. Biopsy showed the microcapsules contained necrotic cells, and were surrounded by a large degree of fibrosis, containing almost no blood vessels (Fig. **9b**). These data suggest that the encapsulated islets were exposed to an inflammatory response shortly after they were transplanted, and that this resulted in the formation of a layer of fibrous tissue blocking the pores on the surface of the microcapsules. The cells inside the microcapsules were effectively deprived of nutrients, and died, perhaps with the exception of a few beta cells.

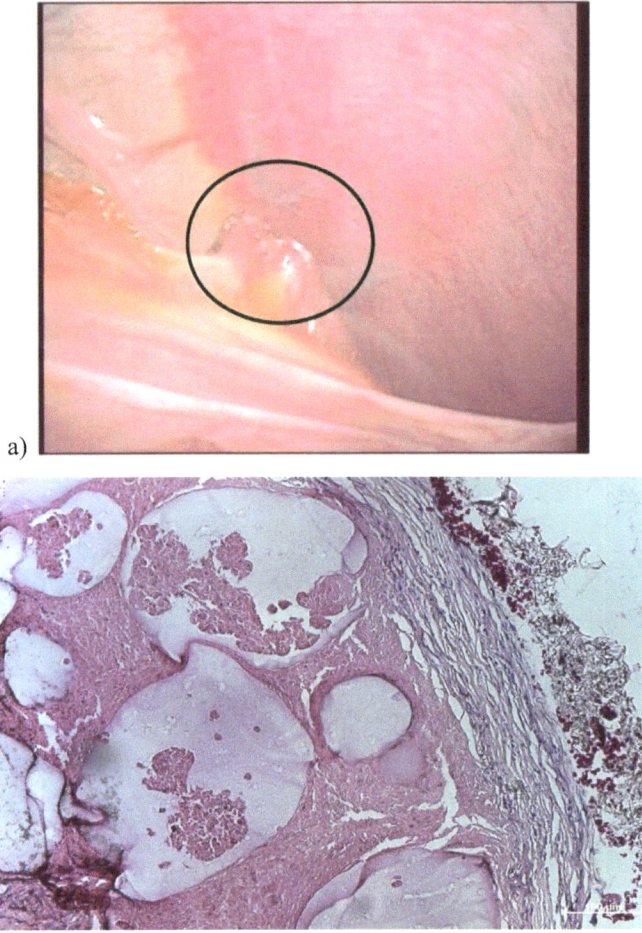

Figure 9: These pictures were taken during laparoscopy 15 months after a person with long standing type 1 diabetes received the first of four encapsulated islet grafts. a) Clusters of encapsulated human islets aggregated together on the superior pole of the spleen. A black circle has been placed around the site to make it easier to identify. b) Necrotic islets inside microcapsules aggregated together and surrounded by relatively avascular fibrous tissue.

That antibodies to glutamic acid decarboxylase were detected in sera suggests that there was antigen leakage from the encapsulated islets into the host, to reactivate the autoimmune process that caused the death of the patients' pancreatic beta cells many years before. This occurred as early as 25 days after a transplant, was detected in 3 recipients and persisted up to at least 2.9 years after being first detected. It is doubtful that this reactivation of autoimmunity would have had any effect on the encapsulated islets, since the cytotoxic T cells causing this phenomenon could not gain entry into the capsules. Likewise, the increase in titre of cytotoxic antibodies in 2 recipients after the infusion of islets is unlikely to have had any adverse effect, even though they may have been able to enter the capsules. The antibodies were IgG in nature with a molecular weight of 150 kDa, which is less than the capsule pore size of 250 kDa. A rise in titre was seen only after day eight post transplantation, by which time insulin secretion had diminished.

Factors which may have stimulated fibrosis in the implanted diabetic humans included the alginate microcapsules or antigens leaking from the encapsulated cells. Previously, we have shown that empty barium alginate microcapsules are not subject to fibrosis when implanted in the peritoneal cavity of immunodeficient and immunocompetent mice [26, 27, 31, 32, 37] and rats [26]. However, when the capsules were implanted into a baboon, fibrosis began within the first week [26], and increased in severity thereafter. The species difference in reactivity presumably relates to immunogenic differences in the recipients. What component of the alginate which leads to immunoreactivity is unclear. The alginate is highly purified by its manufacturer, NovaMatrix/FMC Biopolymer, with few polyphenol or protein contaminants expected. Endotoxin levels are low (< 100 EU/g) and the microcapsules are sterile.

Leaking of antigens of molecular weight smaller than 250 kDa is likely to have been facilitated by the fact that 27% of the encapsulated human islets were not viable (stained red with PI) [14]. However, even fully viable islet preparations would be expected to result in antigen leakage. Indeed, we have observed pericapsular fibrosis when insulin-producing rat cells of viability >95% were allografted into immunocompetent (Wistar) rats [38].

A major outcome of the trial was that there were no major unexpected adverse side effects, such as local or systemic infection after infusion of the encapsulated islets [14]. Perhaps the most noticeable adverse event was nausea in the one recipient who received exenatide, and this eventually required the cessation of the medication. This symptom is a recognized side effect of the drug.

If the use of encapsulated insulin-producing cells is to have an impact clinically as a therapy for type 1 diabetes, two factors need to be addressed. They are enhancing the availability of insulin-producing cells for transplantation, and preventing pericapsular fibrosis.

6. SURROGATE BETA CELLS

Pancreatic progenitors can be derived from human embryonic stem cells [hESC] during a 12 day culture period [39] and when transplanted into mice, will differentiate into mature glucose-responsive beta cells, which will normalize the blood glucose levels of diabetic recipient mice [40]. This *in vivo* development of human pancreatic progenitors when transplanted into immunodeficient mice was described almost 30 years ago by us, the grafted tissue then being from the human fetal pancreas rather than hESC [41, 42]. Using pancreatic progenitors derived from stem cells, which are more readily available than human islets and which do not require the use of pancreases obtained after death, is a logical development. This is especially crucial since the number of people with type 1 diabetes vastly exceeds the number of pancreases available from which islets might be produced. Moreover, the islets when transplanted start to lose their ability to keep recipients normoglycaemic, with almost all being back on exogenous insulin five years after being grafted [4].

Encapsulating pancreatic progenitors, obtained from fetal pigs, and transplanting them into diabetic recipients does result in normalization of blood glucose levels, at least in immunodeficient mice [34]. The progenitors differentiate into mature beta cells over a period of months. Others have shown that human fetal pancreatic tissue placed in a diffusion chamber and implanted in mice also begins to differentiate and lower the blood glucose levels of recipient mice [43]. That encapsulated pancreatic progenitors derived from hESC will function in a similar manner needs to be documented, and experiments have commenced to try and achieve this goal [44]. It is reasonable to believe this will be achieved, as it has been established that hESC placed in microcapsules are capable of differentiating at least into definitive endoderm [45].

A potential disadvantage of transplanting cells derived from hESC is their capacity to form teratomas. Non-encapsulated pancreatic progenitors may contain some pluripotent cells, which will develop into such tumours [40], a reflection that the 12 day differentiation process *in vitro* is not 100% efficient. Results to date show that encapsulation of hESC prevents the formation of teratomas when the encapsulated hESC are transplanted [46], perhaps because of the physical limitations of the capsule. Clinical and regulatory acceptance of this methodology will require the development of adequate controls and quality assurance methods. A supplementary means of preventing the formation of teratomas is to positively select pancreatic progenitors using flow cytometry, now that suitable surface markers, CD200 and CD318, have been described [47].

7. PREVENTING PERICAPSULAR FIBROSIS

Strategies that might be followed to prevent pericapsular fibrosis include:

a) Coating the microcapsules with agents, such as heparin, to reduce the effect of inflammation [38]. This strategy is being used at present in a clinical trial with non-encapsulated human islets infused into the portal vein to reduce the inflammatory process [48] that results in necrosis of a large number of the infused islets.

b) Transplantation of mesenchymal stem cells (MSC) [49]. These cells are advantageous for two reasons. They are hypoimmunogenic because of the absence of class II histocompatibility antigens and co-stimulatory molecules, and low expression of class I histocompatibility antigens [reviewed in 50]. They also have anti-inflammatory properties, based in part on their ability to secrete soluble factors. Indeed, it is because of these properties that MSC are being used in clinical trials to prevent graft *vs.* host disease in bone marrow transplants. Moreover, they have been co-transplanted with islets in rodents and monkeys to enhance the function of the grafts, and reduce/prevent rejection of the tissue from occurring [51].

c) Transplanting the capsules subcutaneously rather than in the peritoneal cavity. Transplanting encapsulated cells in the subcutaneous space result in a reduction of the immunogenic response, as compared to the peritoneal cavity [52]. However, a disadvantage in engrafting cells, such as islets, at this peripheral site is that there is less vascularity than at a more central site, such as in the abdomen [53]. The implantation of islets, which do not function well in poorly vascularised sites because of limited access to oxygen is likely to be a problem, unless strategies to increase angiogenesis are implemented. However, if cells which function well under hypoxic conditions, such as progenitor cells [54], are implanted here, it is reasonable to believe the functional outcomes will be greater.

8. THE FUTURE

With the many developments on the pipeline using encapsulated insulin producing cells as a therapy for diabetes, it can only be a question of time before a reproducible clinical outcome is achieved. In addition to the issues raised elsewhere in this chapter, there are matters of satisfying relevant Regulatory Authorities to ensure the encapsulated cells are safe in addition to being functional. Providing sufficient checks and balances to satisfy the Therapeutic Goods Administration of Australia, or the Food and Drug Administration of the USA, will take some achieving. This is possible as already shown by Geron, who commenced the first clinical trial with cells derived from hESC, for treatment of recent spinal cord lesions, in October 2010. We look forward to the commencement of appropriate clinical trials for the treatment of type 1 diabetes sometime in this decade.

9. STEPWISE PROTOCOLS

9.1. Alginate Based Encapsulation

i)   Carry out the encapsulation procedure using a stainless steel air-driven droplet generator

ii) Remove the islets/cells from culture flasks and pool them together in a 50 ml falcon tube prior to encapsulation procedure.

iii) Wash the islets/cells twice with sterile 0.9 % NaCl followed by centrifugation at 500 rpm for 5 mins to form a pellet and discard the supernatant.

iv) Measure the volume of cell suspension using a 1 ml syringe and calculate the amount of alginate solution required. For 100 μl of islet/cell suspensions add 800 μl of alginate (2.2%) solution (1:8).

v)   Add alginate solution to the cell suspension and mix gently using a 14G catheter. Ensure thorough mixing of alginate and cell suspension to obtain uniform cell distribution within the microcapsules.

vi) Draw 0.8 ml of alginate cell suspension into 1 ml syringe and load onto the encapsulation device.

vii) Securely fix the 1 ml syringe containing alginate-cell suspension onto the encapsulation device.

viii) Set the air flow at 8 L/min and 100 kPa.

ix) Turn on the syringe driver and the plunger in the driver pushes the syringe downwards, thereby forcing the alginate-cell suspension through the encapsulation device to produce alginate microcapsules.

x)   Collect the microcapsules in a sterile 145 mm petri dish containing 30 ml of $BaCl_2$ (20 mM) gelling solution.

xi) Incubate the alginate-cell microcapsules in the $BaCl_2$ solution for 2 min, and wash three times with 0.9 % NaCl to remove excess $BaCl_2$. After repeated washings, allow the microcapsules to settle and discard the supernatant.

xii) Incubate the microencapsulated islets/cells in appropriate supplemented culture media at 37 °C, 5% CO_2 until used for *in vitro* and/or *in vivo* studies.

*Tips to consider

a)   Always filter the 2.2% sodium alginate and $BaCl_2$ solution using a 0.22 μm filter prior to use.

b) Always place the sterile 145 mm petri dish containing 30 ml of $BaCl_2$ gelling solution at a distance of 10 cm from tip of the nozzle of the encapsulation device.

c) Once the alginate cell suspension is made, carry out the encapsulation procedure swiftly to minimize cell death due to hypoxia/starvation.

d) Adjust the air flow rate and pressure to get the desired microcapsules size.

e) It is critical to wash the barium alginate beads at least three times with 0.9% NaCl to remove any excess unbound Ba^{2+} ions.

9.2. Transplantation of Microencapsulated Islets/Insulin Producing Cells into Rodents

i) Perform all surgical procedures within a biosafety cabinet that is UV irradiated prior to use. Sterilize drapes and instruments prior to use.

ii) Induce anaesthesia in mice, for example, with an intraperitoneal injection of pentobarbitone (10 mg/ml) at a dose of 70 mg/kg or 65 mg/kg bodyweight for non-diabetic or diabetic mice respectively.

iii) Place the mouse in a lateral position and spray the incision site with 70 % alcohol.

iv) Make an incision through the skin with a scalpel blade, exposing the subcutaneous tissue and then insert a 14G catheter into the peritoneal cavity.

v) Remove the catheter needle from the peritoneal cavity with only the plastic cannula of the catheter remaining.

vi) Aspirate the encapsulated cells to be transplanted into a 3 ml syringe along with 0.9 % sterile saline and attach to the plastic cannula.

vii) Inject the microcapsules slowly into the peritoneal cavity.

viii) Flush the catheter twice with 0.9 % sterile saline to ensure that all the microcapsules have been transplanted.

ix) Remove the catheter once the microcapsules are injected and suture the peritoneum.

x) Staple the incision site on the skin and place Marcaine (0.05%) on the wound to relieve pain locally.

xi) Place the transplanted animals in a recovery cage and monitor regularly until they are mobile, alert and found to be drinking and eating.

*Tips to consider

a) Administer Buprenorphine (0.07 mg/kg) intra-peritoneal to the animals twice within 24 hrs of surgery to relieve pain. Inject with a further lot of buprenorphine if it seems the mice are in pain after this period.

b) Monitor mice 3 times within the first 24 hours after transplantation and daily for the next 3 days as they tend to lose weight transiently after transplantation.

c) Inject mice with subcutaneous insulin ± intraperitoneal 0.9 % saline if they continue to lose weight and have an elevated blood glucose level.

d) In long term experiments, check mice for development of thymomas and lymphomas, signs of which are shortness of breath, a hunched back and continuing weight loss.

e) Euthanize animals with a weight loss of ≥ 20 % of their pre-transplant body weight.

ACKNOWLEDGEMENTS

We wish to thank all members of the former Diabetes Transplant Unit at the Prince of Wales Hospital/ University of New South Wales who were involved in the numerous experiments carried out with barium alginate microcapsules between 2001 and 2009, when the Unit closed. We are indebted to members of the Chicago Diabetes Project both for supplying human islets and valuable academic contributions. We also wish to thank those in the Australian Diabetes Therapy Project, Biomedical Materials & Devices, at Commonwealth Scientific & Industrial Research Organization for their support in trying to reach a clinical outcome with encapsulated stem cells as a therapy for type 1 diabetes. We are grateful to Drs. Meg Evans and Tim Hughes for critically reviewing this Chapter.

Funding to support the research activities has come from the Australian Foundation for Diabetes Research, Clive & Vera Ramaciotti Foundation, Cooperative Research Centre for Polymers, National Health & Medical Research Council of Australia, National Stem Cell Centre of Australia, the Rebecca L. Cooper Medical Research Foundation and the University of Illinois at Chicago.

CONFLICT OF INTEREST

The author(s) confirm that this chapter content has no conflict of interest.

REFERENCES

[1]   Lacy PE, Kostianovsky M. Method for the isolation of intact islets of Langerhans from the rat pancreas. Diabetes 1967; 16: 35-9.
[2]   Scharp DW, Lacy PE, Santiago JV, McCullough CS, Weide LG, Falqui L, Marchetti P, Gingerich RL, Jaffe AS, Cryer PE *et al.* Insulin independence after islet transplantation into type I diabetic patient. Diabetes 1990; 39: 515-8.
[3]   Shapiro AMJ, Lakey JRT, Ryan EA, Korbutt GS, Toth E, Warnock GL, Kneteman NM, Rajotte R. Islet transplantation in seven patients with type 1 diabetes mellitus using a glucocorticoid-free immunosuppressive regime. N Eng J Med 2000; 343: 230-8.
[4]   CITR, Collaborative Islet Transplant Registry 2009 scientific summary. Available from: www.citregistry.com
[5]   Brendel MD, Hering BJ, Schultz AO, Bretzel RG. International Islet Transplant Registry, Giessen, Germany: University Hospital, 2001: 8.
[6]   International Diabetes Federation. The Diabetes Atlas. 5th Edition. Brussels: International Diabetes Federation; 2011.
[7]   Australian and New Zealand Organ Donor Registry 2011, Excell L, Hee K, Russ G, Eds. Adelaide, South Australia 2011; pp 2-3.
[8]   Haller MJ, Wasserfall CH, McGrail KM, Cintron M, Brusko TM, Wingard JR, Kelly SS, Shuster JJ, Atkinson MA, Schatz DA. Autologous umbilical cord blood transfusion in very young children with type 1 diabetes. Diabetes Care 2009; 32: 2041-6.

[9]   Brands K, Colvin E, Williams LJ, Wang R, Lock RB, Tuch BE. Reduced immunogenicity of first trimester human fetal pancreas. Diabetes 2008; 57: 627-34.

[10]   Buschard K. Cultivation of islets of Langerhans in millipore chamber *in vivo*. Horm Metab Res 1975; 7: 441-2.

[11]   Soon-Shiong P, Heintz RE, Merideth N, Yao QX, Yao Z, Zheng T, Murphy M, Moloney MK, Schmehl M, Harris M, *et al.* Insulin independence in a type 1 diabetic patient after encapsulated islet transplantation. Lancet 1994; 343: 950-1.

[12]   Calafiore R, Basta G, Luca G, Lemmi A, Montanucci MP, Calabrese G, Racanicchi L, Mancuso F, Brunetti P. Microencapsulated pancreatic islet allografts into nonimmunosuppressed patients with type 1 diabetes: first two cases. Diabetes Care 2006; 29: 137-8.

[13]   Basta G, Montanucci P, Luca G, Boselli C, Noya G, Barbaro B, Qi M, Kinzer KP, Oberholzer J, Calafiore R. Long-Term metabolic and immunological follow-up of nonimmunosuppressed patients with type 1 diabetes treated with microencapsulated islet allografts: Four cases. Diabetes Care 2011; 34: 2406-9.

[14]   Tuch BE, Keogh GW, Williams LJ, Wu W, Foster JL, Vaithilingam V, Philips R. Safety and viability of microencapsulated human islets transplanted into humans. Diabetes Care 2009; 32: 1887-9.

[15]   Sun Y, Ma X, Zhou D, Vacek I, Sun AM. Normalization of diabetes in spontaneously diabetic cynomologus monkeys by xenografts of microencapsulated porcine islets without immunosuppression. J Clin Invest 1996; 98: 1417-22.

[16]   Dufrane D, Goebbels RM, Gianello P. Alginate macroencapsulation of pig islets allows correction of streptozotocin-induced diabetes in primates up to 6 months without immunosuppression. Transplantation 2010; 90: 1054-62.

[17]   Elliott RB, Garkavenko O, Tan P, Skaletsky N, Guliev A, Draznin B. Transplantation of microencapsulated neonatal porcine islets in patients with type 1 diabetes: Safety and efficacy. Diabetes 2010; 59 (Suppl 1): A44.

[18]   Schneider S, Feilen PJ, Brunnenmeier F, Minnemann T, Zimmermann H, Zimmermann U, Weber MM. Long-term graft function of adult rat and human islets encapsulated in novel alginate-based microcapsules after transplantation in immunocompetent diabetic mice. Diabetes 2005; 54: 687-93.

[19]   Malavasi NV, Rodrigues DB, Chammas R, Chura-Chambi RM, Barbuto JA, Balduino K, Nonogaki S, Morganti L. Continuous and high-level *in vivo* delivery of endostatin from recombinant cells encapsulated in TheraCyte immunoisolation devices. Cell Transplant 2010; 19: 269-77.

[20]   Maki T, Otsu I, O'Neil JJ, Dunleavy K, Mullon CJ, Solomon BA, Monaco AP. Treatment of diabetes by xenogeneic islets without immunosuppression. Use of a vascularized bioartificial pancreas. Diabetes 1996; 45: 342-7.

[21]   Vaithilingam V, Tuch BE. Islet transplantation and encapsulation: An update on recent developments. Rev Diabet Stud 2011; 8: 63-79.

[22]   van Zanten J, de Vos P. Regulatory considerations in application of encapsulated cell therapies. Adv Exp Med Biol 2010; 70: 1-7.

[23]   Orive G, Hernández RM, Rodríguez Gascón A, Calafiore R, Chang TM, de Vos P, Hortelano G, Hunkeler D, Lacík I, Pedraz JL. History, challenges and perspectives of cell microencapsulation. Trends Biotechnol 2004; 22: 87-92.

[24] Meyer T, Höcht B, Ulrichs K. Xenogeneic islet transplantation of microencapsulated porcine islets for therapy of type I diabetes: long-term normoglycemia in STZ-diabetic rats without immunosuppression. Pediatr Surg Int 2008; 24: 1375-8.

[25] Brissová M, Lacík I, Powers AC, Anilkumar AV, Wang T. Control and measurement of permeability for design of microcapsule cell delivery system. J Biomed Mater Res 1998; 39: 61-70.

[26] Vaithilingam V, Kollarikova G, Qi Meirigeng, Lacik I, Oberholzer J, Guillemin G, Tuch B. Effect of prolonged gelling time on the intrinsic properties of barium alginate microcapsules and its biocompatibility. J Microencapsul 2011; 28: 499-507.

[27] Vaithilingam V, Barbaro B, Oberholzer J, Tuch BE. Functional capacity of human islets after long distance shipment and encapsulation. Pancreas 2011; 40: 247-52.

[28] Tuch BE, Monk RS. Regulation of blood glucose to human levels by human fetal pancreatic xenografts. Transplantation 1991; 51: 1156-60.

[29] Vériter S, Aouassar N, Adnet P-Y, Paridaens M-S, Stuckman C, Jordan B, Karroum O, Gallez B, Gianello P, Dufrane D. The impact of hyperglycemia and the presence of encapsulated islets on oxygenation within a bioartificial pancreas in the presence of mesenchymal stem cells in a diabetic Wistar rat model. Biomaterials 2011; 32: 5945-56.

[30] Vaithilingam V, Quayum N, Joglekar MV, Jensen J, Hardikar AA, Oberholzer J, Guillemin GJ, Tuch BE. Effect of alginate encapsulation on the cellular transcriptome of human islets. Biomaterials 2011; 32: 8416-25.

[31] Vaithilingam V, Oberholzer J, Guillemin GJ, Tuch BE. Beneficial effects of desferrioxamine on encapsulated human islets – *in vitro* & *in vivo* study. Am J Transplant 2010, 10: 1961-9.

[32] Foster JL. PhD Thesis. The microencapsulation and transplantation of fetal pig islet-like cell clusters: A potential therapy for type 1 diabetes, University of New South Wales, 2007.

[33] Vo L, Tuch BE, Wright DC, Keogh GW, Roberts S, Simpson AM, Yao M, Tabiin MT, Valencia SK, Scott H. Lowering of blood glucose to non-diabetic levels in a hyperglycaemic pig by allografting of fetal pig islet-like cell clusters. Transplantation 2001; 71: 1671-7.

[34] Foster JL, Williams G, Williams LJ, Tuch BE. Differentiation of transplanted microencapsulated fetal pancreatic cells. Transplantation 2007; 83: 1440-8.

[35] Tuch BE, Jones A, Turtle JR. Maturation of the response of human fetal pancreatic explants to glucose. Diabetologia 1985; 28: 28-31.

[36] Liu X, Federlin KF, Bretzel RG, Hering BJ, Brendel MD. Persistent reversal of diabetes by transplantation of fetal pig proislets into nude mice. Diabetes 1991; 40: 858-66.

[37] Vaithilingam V, Oberholzer J, Guillemin GJ, Tuch BE. The humanized NOD/SCID mouse as a preclinical model to study the fate of encapsulated human islets. Rev Diabet Stud 2010; 7: 62-73.

[38] Vaithilingam V, Oberholzer J, Lacik I, Larsson R, Guillemin GJ, Tuch BE. Heparinisation of barium alginate microcapsules – *in vitro* & *in vivo* study. Transplantation 2010; 90 (Supp 2): 999.

[39] D'Amour KA, Bang AG, Eliazer S, Kelly OG, Agulnick AD, Smart NG, Moorman MA, Kroon E, Carpenter MK, Baetge EE. Production of pancreatic hormone-expressing endocrine cells from human embryonic stem cells. Nature Biotechnology 2006; 24: 1392-401.

[40] Kroon E, Martinson LA, Kadoya K, Bang AG, Kelly OG, Eliazer S, Young H, Richardson M, Smart NG, Cunningham J, Agulnick AD, D'Amore KA, Carpenter MK, Baetge EE.

Pancreatic endoderm derived from human embryonic stem cells generates glucose-responsive insulin secreting cells *in vivo*. Nature Biotechnology 2008; 26: 443-52.

[41]   Tuch BE, Ng ABP, Jones A, Turtle JR. Histologic differentiation of human fetal pancreatic explants transplanted into nude mice. Diabetes 1984; 33: 1180-7.

[42]   Tuch BE, Osgerby KJ, Turtle JR. Normalization of blood glucose levels in nondiabetic nude mice by human fetal pancreas after induction of diabetes. Transplantation 1988; 46: 608-11.

[43]   Lee SH, Hao E, Savinov AY, Geron I, Strongin AY, Itkin-Ansari P. Human beta-cell precursors mature into functional insulin-producing cells in an immunoisolation device: implications for diabetes cell therapies. Transplantation 2009; 87: 983-91.

[44]   Matveyenko AV, Georgia S, Bhushan A, Butler PC. Inconsistent formation and nonfunction of insulin-positive cells from pancreatic endoderm derived from human embryonic stem cells in athymic nude rats. Am J Physiol Endocrinol Metab 2010; 299: E713-20.

[45]   Chayosumrit M, Tuch B, Sidhu K. Alginate microcapsule for propagation and directed differentiation of hESCs to definitive endoderm. Biomaterials 2010; 31: 505-14.

[46]   Dean SK, Yulyana, Williams G, Sidhu KS, Tuch BE. Differentiation of encapsulated embryonic stem cells after transplantation. Transplantation 2006; 82: 1175-84.

[47]   Kelly OG, Chan MY, Martinson LA, Kadoya K, Ostertag TM, Ross KG, Richardson M, Carpenter MK, D'Amour KA, Kroon E, Moorman M, Baetge EE, Bang AG. Cell-surface markers for the isolation of pancreatic cell types derived from human embryonic stem cells. Nat Biotech 2011; 29: 750-6.

[48]   Cabric S, Sanchez J, Lundgren T, Foss A, Felldin M, Källen R, Salmela K, Tibell A, Tufveson G, Larsson R, Korsgren O, Nilsson B. Islet surface heparinization prevents the instant blood-mediated inflammatory reaction in islet transplantation. Diabetes 2007; 56, 2008–15.

[49]   Vaithilingam V, Bean P, McFarland G, Evans MD, Tuch BE. Co-encapsulation of mesenchymal stem cells reduces pericapsular fibrotic overgrowth in a xenotransplantation setting. Aust Soc Stem Cell Res 2011; 4: 50-1 (A85).

[50]   Chen FH, Tuan RS. Mesenchymal stem cells in arthritic diseases. Arthritis Res Ther 2008; 10: 223-34.

[51]   Berman DM, Willman MA, Han D, Kleiner G, Kenyon NM, Cabrera O, Karl JA, Wiseman, RW, O'Connor DH, Bartholomew AM, Kenyon NS. Mesenchymal stem cells enhance allogeneic islet engraftment in nonhuman primates. Diabetes 2010; 59: 2558-68.

[52]   Dufrane D, van Steenberghe M, Goebbels R-M, Saliez A, Guiot Y, Gianello P. The influence of implantation site on the biocompatibility and survival of alginate encapsulated pig islets in rats. Biomaterials 2006; 27: 3201-8.

[53]   Vériter S, Aouassar N, Adnet P-Y, Paridaens M-S, Stuckman C, Jordan B, Karroum O, Gallez B, Gianello P, Dufrane D. The impact of hyperglycemia and the presence of encapsulated islets on oxygenation within a bioartificial pancreas in the presence of mesenchymal stem cells in a diabetic Wistar rat model. Biomaterials 2011; 32: 5945-56.

[54]   Bae D, Mondragon-Teran P, Hernandez D, Ruban L, Mason C, Bhattacharya SS, Veraitch FS. Hypoxia enhances the generation of retinal progenitor cells from human induced pluripotent and embryonic stem cells. Stem Cells Dev 2012; 21: 1344-55.

Send Orders of Reprints at reprints@benthamscience.net

CHAPTER 3

The Diversity of Uses for Cellulose Sulphate Encapsulation

John A. Dangerfield[1,*], Brian Salmons[1], Randolph Corteling[2], Jean-Pierre Abastado[3], John Sinden[2], Walter H. Gunzburg[1] and Eva M. Brandtner[1,4]

[1]*SG Austria Pte Ltd/Austrianova Singapore Pte Ltd, Biopolis, Singapore;* [2]*ReNeuron Group Plc, Guildford, Surrey, England;* [3]*Singapore Immunology Network (SIgN), Biopolis, Singapore and* [4]*VIVIT Molecular Biology Laboratory, Dornbirn, Austria*

Abstract: In this chapter we propose sodium cellulose sulphate (SCS) as a prime candidate for clinical application of encapsulated cells and present data for uses of SCS encapsulation for the direct delivery of therapeutic antibodies and advanced approaches for stem cell therapy. We also provide a simple lab protocol allowing researchers to make capsules at the bench without the need for expensive machinery.

Keywords: Live cell encapsulation, bioencapsulation, sodium cellulose sulphate, therapeutic antibodies, biomolecule release, long-term release, long-term survival, stem cells, biocompatibility, GMP manufacturing, immune protection, patient safety, storage capability, localisation, removability.

1. INTRODUCTION

The treatment of diseases and disorders by microencapsulation of living cells and the subsequent implantation of these capsules into patients were pioneered 30 years ago [1]. It can be considered as a specialised type of cell therapy and one that is potentially safer since the cells are physically separated from the body as well as more efficacious since the cells are confined to the site at which they are implanted and have the potential to be removed if necessary after treatment is complete.

Alginate was one of the first materials used to encapsulate cells and this seaweed derived material is still in use today, mainly in the development of encapsulated

Address correspondence to John A. Dangerfield: Austrianova Singapore Pte Ltd, 20 Biopolis Way, #05-518 Centros, Singapore; Tel: +65 6779 2932; Fax: +65 6774 5569; E-mail: dangerfield@sgaustria.com

cell treatments for diabetes (see chapters 1 and 2). More recently, subseive agarose beads have also been used for cell encapsulation (see chapter 6).

We have focussed on the use of sodium cellulose sulphate (SCS) as a cell encapsulation material [2, 3]. Capsules consisting of polymers of SCS and polydiallyldimethyl ammonium chloride (pDADMAC) offer a number of advantages including:

- ability to reproducibly source, produce and characterise the SCS starting material.

- robustness of the capsules (permitting delivery through needles or catheters without bursting).

- good biocompatibility for the cells in the microcapsule.

- cells like to grow and survive for extended periods in the capsule but they do not escape due to a three dimensional contact inhibition.

- good biocompatibility and inertness of the capsules when implanted at various sites in the body.

- lack of an immune or inflammatory response either to the capsule material or to the cells that are protected by it.

- lack of fibrous overgrowth.

- large scale GMP manufacturing of an encapsulated cell medicinal product has been achieved [4].

- ability to freeze the encapsulated cells and thus store and ship them.

We have developed the SCS encapsulation technology originally for the treatment of solid tumours such as pancreatic cancer and breast. These encapsulated cells were tested in clinical trials and shown to be both efficacious and (perhaps more importantly when considering other uses of the technology) safe when they remain in the body for at least two years [5, 6].

Consequently, and building on the clinical data we already have with SCS encapsulated cells, we have been encapsulating various cells types in order to design therapies for the treatment of a wide variety of diseases with various partners. Some of these approaches to treat diseases such as virus infections, tumours and improved stem cell treatments are discussed in this article.

2. RELEASE OF ANTIBODIES FROM ENCAPSULATED CELLS

2.1. General Considerations: Immune Protection

The main purpose of cell encapsulation is to protect the cells from the immune system. The capsules act as a mechanical barrier between the encapsulated cells and their surroundings. This is accomplished by the capsule wall which has pores that are big enough to allow nutrients to diffuse in and waste products out of the capsules and of course is permissive for the release of the therapeutic molecule of interest. On the other hand, the pores are small enough to deny access to immune cells like macrophages, neutrophils and T-cells.

For release of antibodies from encapsulated cells the membrane pores must, of course, be large enough to allow the passage of antibodies. Therefore, for *in-vivo* application of this technology the question presents itself whether (a) antibodies from the host can get into the capsules and (b) if this could result in immune rejection of the encapsulated cells.

The answer to the first question (a) is yes, there is no reason why antibodies could not get into the capsules since they can get out and the mechanism of crossing the capsule membrane is a passive one. However, there are several reasons why this does not result in immune rejection of the encapsulated cells. Firstly, the concentration gradient favours the exit of antibodies from the capsules since the production of antibodies by the encapsulated cells leads to a high local concentration of antibodies inside the capsules, much higher than in the surrounding tissue. This means although, in theory, traffic can occur in both directions, antibodies diffuse out of the capsules much more efficiently than into the capsules.

Secondly (b), for an immune rejection to occur, antibodies of the right specificity must be present. Antibodies are secreted by mature B-cells which evolve from naive B-cells after contact with the antigen that their receptor is specific for. After activation of the B-cells, a cascade of events happens which involves the expansion of the respective B-cell clone and results in a large number of mature B-cells, so called plasma cells, which are able to secrete antibodies. Since the initial step requires cell to cell contact between the naive B-cell and the surface antigen on the encapsulated cells and the capsules do not allow cell to cell contact across their membrane, activation of the specific B-cells should not happen. This means, although antibodies can in principle enter the capsules, there is no specific humoral immune response against the encapsulated cells.

However, in the unlikely case that a capsule breaks and cells are exposed, as well as in a xenotransplantation scenario where natural antibodies (antibodies which are present in higher primates independent of prior infection or vaccination) come into play, the presence of antibodies with affinity to the cells inside the capsules cannot be ruled out. But even in this latter case the encapsulated cells are still protected. Antibodies do not attack and kill cells as such. They just earmark them for further attention from other players in the immune system. There are two ways in which foreign cells are eliminated from the body once they are marked with antibodies. One is *via* effector cells and requires cell to cell contact. In the case of encapsulated cells, this is prevented by the capsule wall. The other way is *via* the classical pathway of complement activation and requires a high concentration of antibodies bound to the surface of the target cell. Proteins of the complement system, prior to activation, are part of large multi protein complexes which cannot enter the capsules. For example, the first step of the classical pathway involves the C1 complex. C1 binds to antibody molecules which are attached to antigens (resulting in immune complexes) and thereby initiates the cascade. With a size of 766 kDa the C1 complex is too large to enter the capsules. The same is true for other complement protein complexes involved in the other steps of complement activation. Therefore, encapsulated antibody producing cells are protected from the action of the complement system as well as from the access of effector cells. The experimental data presented below confirm that, indeed, encapsulated hybridoma cells can survive *in vivo* for prolonged periods of time.

2.2. Applications of Antibody Production from Encapsulated Cells

2.2.1. Depletion of Immune Cell Lineages

The biological role of different immune cell lineages can be studied by depleting the cell lineage of interest and looking at the effect in animal models. Depletion of individual lineages can be achieved by using cytotoxic antibodies against surface markers on the target cells. Such antibodies are available for the depletion of CD4+ and CD8+ T cells [7-18], granulocytes [19-21], CD20+ B cells [22, 23] for example.

For sustained depletion standard protocols see the animals being injected with antibodies several times per week. The treatment as such is costly and labour intensive. Therefore, release of the antibodies from encapsulated cells within the body is an attractive alternative. Once implanted into the body, encapsulated cells can survive and produce antibody in constant amounts over sustained periods of time. This avoids the "peaks and troughs" of antibody concentration which occurs as a result of infusion or injection of the large amounts necessary to sustain the effect until the next infusion is made. These large quantities are also associated with negative immune-related stimulation, causing faster clearance of the antibodies and for some antibodies anti-idiotypic responses, and so the effects of the antibodies decrease with time. The constant low amount released from the capsules avoids this scenario. This has been demonstrated in a proof-of concept study in which a rat hybridoma producing a cytotoxic anti-mouse CD8 antibody (2.43) [7] was encapsulated and implanted in mice (Fig. **1**). The capsules containing the 2.43 antibody producing cells were retrieved from the mice 8 weeks after implantation and shown to still retain viability. Thus even in a xenogeneic setting, encapsulation protects cells from immune attack (Fig. **2**).

These findings indicate that the long-term depletion of immune cell lineages using encapsulated antibody producing cells is feasible and warrants further optimisation.

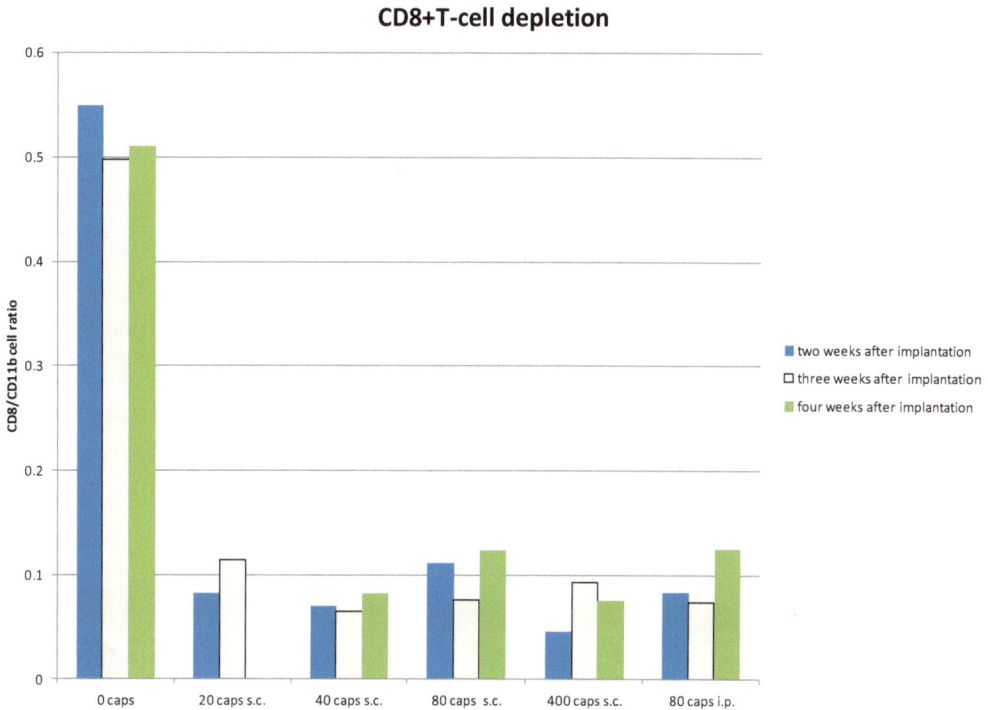

Figure 1: CD8+ T-cell depletion in mice implanted with encapsulated cells producing 2.43 antibody. The amount of CD8+ T-cells in the peripheral blood of mice was measured in relation to the amount of CD11b cells, which are not affected by the treatment. CD8+/CD11b+ cell ratios are shown for mice implanted with 0, 20, 40, 80, 400 capsules subcutaneously (s.c.) and 80 capsules intraperitoneally (i.p.). Animal care and experimental procedures were approved by the Institutional Animal Care and Use Committee (IACUC) (Application No. 090425) of the Biological Resource Center, 20 Biopolis Way, Singapore 138668.

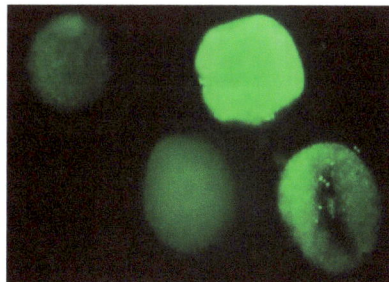

Figure 2: Encapsulated rat cells are still alive eight weeks after implantation into the body of immunocompetent mice. Encapsulated cells were removed from the body of a mouse eight weeks after implantation, stained with calcein-AM, an indicator for living cells and visualised by fluorescence microscopy. Animal care and experimental procedures were approved by the Institutional Animal Care and Use Committee (IACUC) (Application No. 090425) of the Biological Resource Center, 20 Biopolis Way, Singapore 138668.

2.2.2. Encapsulation of mAb Producing Cells for the Treatment of Infectious Disease

FrCas E is a chimeric virus consisting of mouse ectopic retrovirus CasBrE (clone 15-1) env and 3' pol sequences in a Friend murine leukemia virus (FMuLV) background. FrCasE virus infection in new-born mice is an ideal animal model of infectious disease since it causes a clear phenotype, *i.e.* rapidly progressing neurodegenerative disease which is fatal within 6 weeks, with 100% incidence. This model was used to show that neutralising antibody released from encapsulated hybridoma cells is able to rescue a large percentage of the animals even in a non-optimised first experiment [24]. This was the case irrespective of whether the capsules were implanted concurrently with viral infection (80% survival of the treated animals) or 2 days after the infection (65% survival of the treated animals) (Fig. **3**) which strongly indicates potential use in a therapeutic rather than just prophylactic setting.

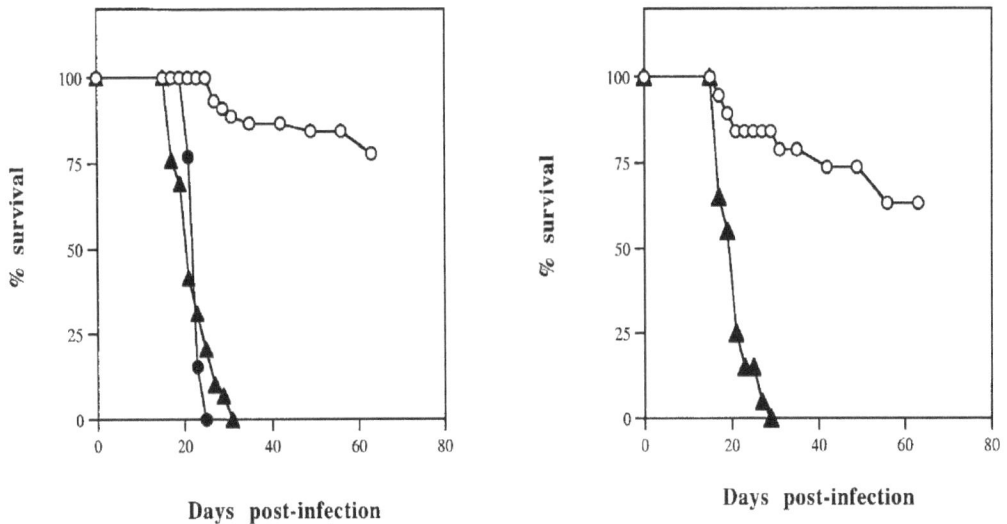

Figure 3: Survival of FrCasE-infected mice treated with 667 cell-containing capsules [24]. (Left) Four-day-old mice were infected by intraperitoneal injection with 5 x 10^4 focus forming units (FFU). Twenty-nine mice received no further treatment (full triangles). G8P2B5 (control antibody; full circles) and 667 (FrCasE neutralising antibody; open circles) hybridoma cell-containing cellulose sulphate capsules were subcutaneously implanted in 13 and 45 mice, respectively, on the day of infection. (Right) Twenty 4-day-old mice infected with 5 x 10^4 FrCasE FFU received no further treatment (full triangle) and a further 20 infected mice received 667 cell-containing capsules on day 2 post-infection (open circle), respectively. Figure taken from published article [24].

This goes to show that encapsulated antibody producing cells are a means to fight infectious disease and potentially protect the body in the critical time window between exposures to a pathogen and evolving of the body's own adaptive immune response.

Besides *in vivo* use, encapsulation of antibody or antibody like producing cells can be of great interest for the industrial production of antibodies by the biotech industry. The capsules can act as a pre-filtration device and eliminate cost-intensive steps during downstream processing of antibody products. Such encapsulated products should be seen favourably by industry since they may allow for new IP surrounding old technologies in combination with capsules. This may allow generation of new patents or extension of old patents, something it can be assumed is much needed when looking at the current portfolios of many of the large pharmaceutical companies.

Treatments with therapeutic antibodies come at costs of at least US$ 40,000 per year per patient (Table **1**). Worldwide, the market for therapeutic antibodies has a volume of over US$ 50 billion. Patients need frequent injections, sometimes for their entire life. There is tremendous potential in finding more cost-efficient ways of delivery for these therapeutic antibodies. The encapsulation and subsequent implantation of the cells producing these antibodies opens a whole new range of possibilities and makes such therapies more accessible and affordable for a vast number of patients.

Table 1: Therapeutic antibodies for the treatment of cancer

Antibody	Trade Name	Target	Type	Indication	Approval
Rituximab	Rituxan® Mabthera®	CD20	chimeric	non-Hodgkin lymphoma	1997
Trastuzumab	Herceptin®	ErbB2	humanised	breast cancer	1998
Gemtuzumab Ozogamicin	Mylotarg®	CD33	humanised	acute myelogeneous leukemia	2000
Alemtuzumab	Campath®	CD52	humanised	chronic lmphocytic leukemia	2001
Ibritumomab Tiuxetan	Zevalin®	CD20	murine	non-Hodgkin lymphoma	2002

Table 1: cont....

Tositumomab	Bexxar®	CD20	murine	non-Hodgkin lymphoma	2003
Bevacizumab	Avastin®	VEGF	humanised	colorectal cancer	2004
Panitumumab	Vectibix®	EGFR	human	colorectal cancer	2006
Ofatumamab	Arzerra®	CD20	human	chronic lmphocytic leukemia	2009
Brentuximab Vedotin	Adcetris®	CD30	chimeric	large cell lymphoma and Hodgkin lymphoma	2011
Ipilimumab	Yervoy®	CTLA-4	human	melanoma	2011
Cetuximab	Erbitux®	EGFR	chimeric	colorectal cancer head and neck cancer	2004 2006

3. HOW ENCAPSULATION CAN HELP THE BUDDING STEM CELL INDUSTRY

3.1. Is There a Budding Stem Cell Industry?

Before considering the reasons for wanting to encapsulate stem cells, it is firstly important to decide if stem cells have lived up to their expectations in terms of medical potential, *i.e.* does it makes sense to pursue such applications? Some may consider that stem cell progress has been slower than predicted, attributable most likely to the long lasting media hype, but there are some marked examples which suggest that the answer to this question could indeed be "yes".

2012 has seen the world's first, market approved, allogeneic cell therapy products. The product CARTISTEM® from the Korean biotech company Medipost Co. Ltd. was approved for sale in Korea by the Korean FDA in January 2012. Their product is manufactured using mesenchymal stem cells (MSC), which are also known as mesenchymal precursor cells (MPC) which, in Medipost's case, are extracted from publicly donated umbilical cord blood. Sales are taking off in Korea for the use of CARTISTEM® as an off-the-shelf product to treat degenerative arthritis and knee cartilage defects. It is currently in further clinical trials under guidance of the FDA and is expected to be approved for sale in the U.S. before 2014. Medipost also has three other products in human trials based on the same cells which they claim can be used for the treatment of neuro-degenerative disorders such as Alzheimer's, pulmonary disorders such as bronchopulmonary dysplasia and the transplant engraftment disorder, graft *vs.* host disease (Table **2**). In May 2012 the U.S. based company Osiris Therapeutics Inc. also claimed to be the world's first company to receive market clearance for an approved stem cell drug called Prochymal[TM]. Osiris also has several other late stage trials going on with their MPC-based products Prochymal[TM] and Chongrogen[TM] which offer hope to children suffering from the life threatening graft *vs.* host disease as well as those with Crohn's disease and a number of pulmonary related problems such as emphysema and bronchitis (Table **2**).

Table 2: World-wide clinical trials using allogeneic stem cell based therapeutics (as of July 2012). Information sources include the U.S. governmental National Institutes of Health website (http://clinicaltrials.gov/ct2/home), the websites of the companies as well as other media sources. In many cases, information between company websites and the government database was conflicting. Mostly, the company websites suggested trials were further along. Although this may be factual, in these cases, the government database information was used. Trials at various enrolment or pre-recruitment stages, trials which were terminated or trials for which information has not been updated within the past two years were not included. Trials are listed alphabetically based on the sponsor's name.

Sponsor (Company Location)	Indication(s)	Technology/Product	Status
Advanced Cell Technology Inc. (USA)	Stargardt's Macular Dystrophy	human embryonic stem cell derived retinal pigmented epithelial (MA09-hRPE) cells	Phase I/II (ongoing)
Advanced Cell Technology (USA)	Dry Age-Related Macular Degeneration	human embryonic stem cell derived retinal pigmented epithelial (MA09-hRPE) cells	Phase I/II (ongoing)
Geron Corp. (USA)	Spinal Cord Injury	human embryonic stem cells (GRNOPC1)	Phase I (ongoing)
MEDIPOST Co. Ltd. (Korea)	Cartilage Injury		
Osteoarthritis	human umbilical cord blood derived-mesenchymal stem cells/CARTISTEM®	Phase III (completed)	

Table 2: cont....

MEDIPOST Co. Ltd. (Korea)	Dementia of the Alzheimer's Type	human umbilical cord blood derived-mesenchymal stem cells/NEUROSTEM®	Phase I (completed)
MEDIPOST Co. Ltd. (Korea)	Acute Leukemia	human umbilical cord blood derived-mesenchymal stem cells	Phase I/II (completed)
MEDIPOST Co. Ltd. (Korea)	Bronchopulmonary Dysplasia	human umbilical cord blood derived-mesenchymal stem cells/PNEUMOSTEM®	Phase I (completed)
MEDIPOST Co. Ltd. (Korea)	Graft-*vs.*-Host Disease	human umbilical cord blood-derived mesenchymal stem cells	Phase I/II (recruiting)
Mesoblast Ltd. (Australia)	Degenerative Disc Disease in Subjects with Chronic Discogenic Lumbar Back Pain	adult human mesenchymal precursor cells (MPCs) with hyaluronic acid carrier	Phase II (recruiting)
Mesoblast Ltd. (Australia)	Degenerative Disc Disease in Subjects requiring Lumbar Interbody Infusion	adult human mesenchymal precursor cells (MPCs)/NeoFuse^{TM} combined with MasterGraft® matrix fusion granules	Phase II (ongoing)
Mesoblast Ltd. (Australia)	Cervical Degenerative Disc Disease in Subjects Undergoing Multi-Level Anterior Cervical Discectomy	adult human mesenchymal precursor cells (MPCs)/NeoFuse^{TM} combined with MasterGraft® matrix fusion granules	Phase II (ongoing)
Mesoblast Ltd. (Australia)	Degenerative Disc Disease in Subjects Requiring Posterolateral Lumbar Fusion (PLF)	adult human mesenchymal precursor cells (MPCs)/NeoFuse^{TM} combined with MasterGraft® matrix fusion granules	Phase I/II (ongoing)
Mesoblast Ltd. (Australia)	Anterior Cruciate Ligament Injury/Osteoarthritis	adult human mesenchymal precursor cells (MPCs, MSB-	Phase I/II (recruiting)

		CAR001) with hyaluronic acid carrier	

Table 2: cont....

Mesoblast Ltd. (Australia)	Type 2 Diabetes	adult human mesenchymal precursor cells (MPCs)	Phase I/II (recruiting)
Osiris Therapeutics Inc. (USA)	Treatment-refractory Crohn's Disease	adult human mesenchymal stem cells/PROCHYMAL™	Phase III (completed)
Osiris Therapeutics Inc. (USA)	Recovery Following Partial Medial Meniscectomy	adult human mesenchymal stem cells/Chondrogen™	Phase I/II (completed)
Osiris Therapeutics Inc. (USA)	Moderate to Severe Chronic Pulmonary Disease/Pulmonary Emphysema/Chronic Bronchitis	adult human mesenchymal stem cells/PROCHYMAL™	Phase II (completed)
Osiris Therapeutics Inc. (USA)	Treatment-refractory (1) and Newly Diagnosed (2) Acute Graft *vs*. Host Disease	(1) and (2): varying doses of adult human mesenchymal stem cells/PROCHYMALTM (2): in combination with corticosteroids	(1) Phase II (completed) (2)Phase III (completed)
ReNeuron Limited (UK)	Stable Ischemic Stroke	neural stem cells (CTX0E03)	Phase I (ongoing)
Stempeutics Research Pvt. Ltd. Stempcutics Research Malaysia SDN. BHD. (India/Malaysia)	Osteoarthritis of the Knee Joint	Bone marrow derived adult mesenchymal stem cells/Stempeucel - CLI™	Phase II (recruiting)
Stempeutics Research Pvt. Ltd. (India)	Critical Limb Ischemia due to Buerger's Disease	Bone marrow derived adult mesenchymal stem cells/Stempeucel - CLI™	Phase II (recruiting)

There are other stem cell companies with allogeneic products in various stages of clinical trials as well. Until recently, the U.S. biotech Geron Corporation has used human embryonic stem cells (HSC) as a platform and has undertaken a Phase I study in patients with thoracic spinal cord injuries (Table **2**). They also have evidence for therapeutic benefit of their HSC-based products in the areas of heart muscle regeneration, diabetes, cartilage repair and development of cancer vaccines. ReNeuron Group Plc. in U.K. has a neural based stem cell line in ongoing Phase I for the treatment of stroke (Table **2**). But possibly the most advanced and financially endowed stem cell company currently is Mesoblast Ltd. in Australia, who has ongoing trials in four disease areas, including a recent successful Phase II outcome and permission to begin a Phase III. Their cell technology platform is based on MPC derived from bone marrow aspirates as well as other tissues of healthy adults and they have good evidence showing potential for the treatment of cardiovascular diseases foremost but also diabetes, bone and cartilage repair and replacement and some forms of eye disease (Table **2**).

Advanced Cell Technology (ACT) is performing two trials with HSC aimed at improving the vision of patients with Stargardt's Macular Dystrophy and Dry Age-Related Macular Degeneration (Table **2**). Patients' eyes were injected with retinal pigmented epithelial cells derived from human embryonic stem cells. The preliminary findings appear to be promising, as judged by the outcomes from two patients treated as part of the trial. During the trial, neither patient's vision worsened nor were there obvious negative side effects [25].

3.2. Reasons for Encapsulating Stem Cells

When discussing the encapsulation of stem cells, it is often asked, "How can it work because the stem cells are trapped inside the capsule?" This question exists because of the common misconception that implanted stem cells grow, differentiate and/or develop to become the regenerated tissue and that the presence of this tissue itself is necessary to have the therapeutic effect. Although this may be true for a few special cases, it is now generally accepted amongst experts that the vast majority of stem cells react on implantation to their micro-environment to release a wide array of soluble factors that mediate beneficial paracrine effects and may greatly contribute to the therapeutic effect. These include cytokines, growth factors and microvesicles which then act locally to trigger the patient's own systems into repair [26].

Mesoblast, for example, clearly states this to be the case on their website under the technology section, "The MPCs act as micro-drug factories providing the secretion of trophic factors that then exert multiple mechanisms of action including but not limited to anti-apoptosis (anti-death) of cells, regeneration of damaged tissue, recruitment of the body's own tissue specific precursor cells and proliferation/inhibition of relevant cells types including blood vessels". This is now accepted in the field of stem cell research, as well as industry, to be the main mechanism of action for stem cells [27].

This in turn means that most, if not all, of these mechanisms can still work when the cells are in an encapsulated state since the factors will be released through the semi-permeable outer-membrane of the capsule. Recently data was gathered using a commercial, clinically approved, stem cell line to show encapsulating stem cells in polymers of sodium cellulose sulphate can work well on several different levels. Most, if not all, are sensitive to their environment, therefore, initially growth and survival were tested (Fig. **4**). Since basic encapsulation in cellulose sulphate was not a problem for the growth and survival of this stem cell line, the morphology of the cells was monitored once released from the capsules. Stem cells that have been grown inside capsules for several weeks were morphologically the same as non-encapsulated cells grown under standard, optimised conditions (Fig. **5**). Interestingly, inside the capsules, the cells from this neural based line migrated towards each other to form neuro-spheres as would be expected under the 3-dimensional conditions which the capsule provides (Fig. **5B**). Taken together, this was a strong indication that the cells had maintained their pre-encapsulation characteristics.

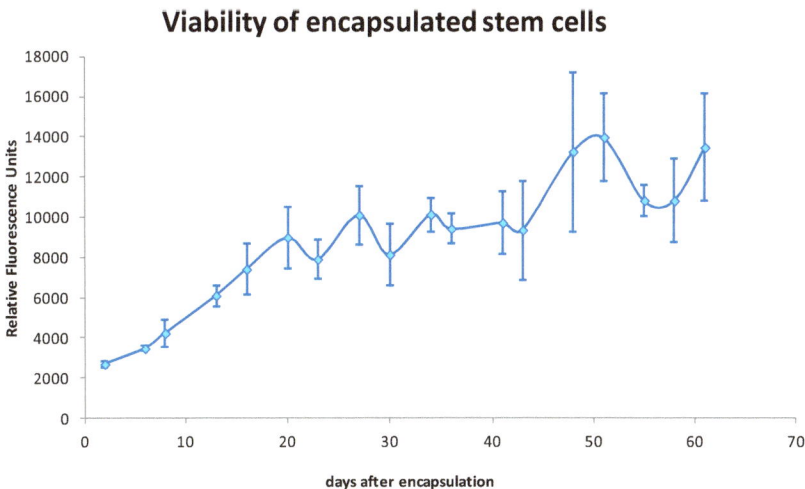

Figure 4: Long term survival of encapsulated stem cells. A clinically approved stem cell line showed growth and survival for over sixty days when encapsulated using polymers of sodium cellulose sulphate.

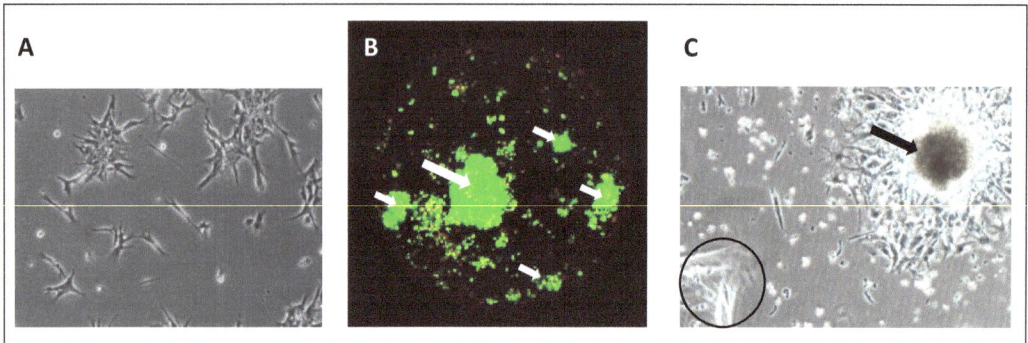

Figure 5: Morphology of neural stem cells is maintained after sodium cellulose sulphate encapsulation. **(A)** Cells cultured under conditions for normal maintenance, viewed with standard light microscopy. **(B)** Live/dead staining viewed with fluorescence microscopy show as indicated by white arrows that cells grow and migrate towards each other inside the capsule to form neuro-spheres of increasing size. Green indicates living cells and red dead or dying cells. **(C)** Cells after the capsule has been dissolved away *in vitro*, viewed with standard light microscopy. A dissolved capsule fragment is indicated by the circle. A neuro-sphere is indicated with the black arrow. Cells growing away from the neuro-sphere have the same morphology as non-encapsulated cells in (A).

Having established that there are many medically interesting stem cells and that they would in principal still function normally when encapsulated, the final and most critical point to address is the reason or benefit to encapsulating them. Despite their multi-tiered use in humans already, many understand there are some serious concerns and challenges still to be overcome. These can be divided into two main categories; one being safety concerns from authorities, regulators, scientists and companies alike about the fate of the cells after implantation (reviewed in [28]) and the other being issues relating to the sensitivity of cell growth, upscaling and general manufacturing procedures (reviewed in [29]). Encapsulation can provide solutions in all these areas as well as provide other benefits which will be discussed below.

Concerning the fate of the cells and the safety implications this has. Some years back it was discovered in animal models that stem cells can differentiate into tissue with tumorigenic capability and from a type of tumour called a teratoma [30]. Since then, similar incidents of malignant outgrowth from stem cells have been recorded by others [31-33]. In addition to the 500 or so companies that can be found in the internet dealing with so called stem cell products (with varying levels of seriousness), many patients have also been treated with autologous stem cells at clinics all round the world. All such treatments are not approved through regulatory bodies although most large hospitals have such autologous programmes running. So the teratoma and other malignant outgrowth findings did not prevent stem cells being implanted into patients and there have been some worrying and notable cases as a result. For example there was a brain tumour in a boy with ataxia telangiectasia that was treated with stem cells. The tumour cells were shown to be of non-host origin, suggesting strongly that it was derived from the transplanted neural stem cells [34], and there have been other cases where adverse effects and growths have been shown after stem cell treatments [35, 36]. If the cells had been implanted in stable capsules, it is likely that none of these incidences would have occurred.

Despite many attempts to study cell fate in animal models, even in the case of the approved product CARTISTEM®, it is not known what happens to the implanted cells in human patients. This is because there are no available technologies allowing stem cells to be marked for tracking purposes without detrimentally affecting the cells. Both external labelling with antibody tags, internal marking with fluorescent particles, or genetic marking by introducing a gene such as the green fluorescent protein for example, all result in various changes to the cell. This can manifest as damage the therapeutic potential since most stem cells are very sensitive to any manipulation causing them to change, usually for the worse. The change could also for example cause an increase in immunogenicity, *i.e.* making the cells have a higher profile to the patient's immune system because of the added foreign components, meaning they are cleared before being able to carry out their therapeutic function. It must also be considered that any such changes provide additional hurdles from a regulatory perspective since any new components to the product need to be approved for human use. Taken together, this means that within the entire field, still only theories and speculation exists as to the fate of stem cells once implanted in human patients. For interest's sake alone, most commonly it's proposed that they undergo apoptosis (since this would be convenient) or that they migrate away from the site of implantation.

Encapsulation of the cells could have prevented the severe adverse events and could entirely address the above discussed concerns since the cells are not released from the capsules at any stage after implantation. It should also make it easier for companies to gain permission for clinical trials and allow companies, hospitals and clinics alike a considerable measure of safety when undertaking such procedures. Another benefit of having cells in capsules is that they hold the cells at the locality of treatment. It is not known how long naked cells stay at the desired site. It is known however that many implanted cells have a high tendency for migration *in vivo*. There is evidence to suggest that implanted cells wander away from the implantation site quite quickly, between hours and days depending on the cells and site of implantation [37, 38]. Encapsulation clearly allows the possibility to keep the cells at the site of implantation since typically capsules are around 1 mm in size and contain thousands of cells each, so they remain physically fixed at the site. For example, this would be true for sub-cutaneous, intra-muscular, brain, peri-organ or peri-tumoral application but not the case for inter-peritoneal application or injection into the blood system, where the capsules would move around. Having them around at the desired location for longer period may well enhance their therapeutic effect. Encapsulation can also improve treatment efficacy by enhancing the length of time that stem cells can survive *in vivo*. If capsules are implanted sub-cutaneous, this also offers the possibility of removal of the cells after treatment is complete, since they can be found easily later at the same place they were implanted. This is important since many patients are concerned about having foreign cells in them for the rest of their time.

Finally, although most claim that allogeneic stem cells are non-immunogenic, this is still not fully understood. It certainly seems that they are less immunogenic, than for example a syngeneic somatic cell line would be, however, it may be that immune system plays a role in the fate or pre-mature clearance of implanted stem cells. Again, encapsulation would prevent this, since cells of the patient's immune system cannot enter the capsules.

Encapsulation also has several potential benefits for manufacturing. The vast majority of stem cells are cultured in monolayer system as opposed to stirred reactors which makes upscaling highly manpower and materials intensive. This is one of the major barriers to making large volume, off-the-shelf stem cell products and is in turn why many of the large pharma companies are holding back on development of stem cell products until these issues are solved. It's proving very difficult to evolve stem cells into growth in bioreactors since generally speaking they are highly sensitive to all kinds of manipulation, including physical stress, meaning that stemness of the cells is not maintained under stirred conditions. Having cells inside capsules can entirely circumvent this problem and allow monolayer dependent growth under stirred conditions since the inside of capsule acts as a substrate for the cells to attach and the outside of the capsule acts as a protective device against collisions with other capsules and sheer stresses of the vortex caused by stirring. Bioreactor benefits, such as increased oxygen availability, reduction in plastic consumables, ease of changing of culture medium and harvesting of the product can be then be gained for stem cells.

Capsules may be dissolved *in vitro* prior to use in order to release the cells or implanted directly as capsules into the patient, depending on the application. The cellulose sulphate encapsulation technology Cell-in-a-Box® developed by the company SG Austria Pte Ltd/Austrianova Singapore Pte Ltd in Singapore allows for cryopreservation of capsules containing cells [4]. Frozen capsules can be stored for many months without appreciable loss of cell viability; an attribute that makes cellulose sulphate desirable over other more commonly used encapsulation technologies such as alginate which cannot be frozen (Fig. **6**). This attribute has a

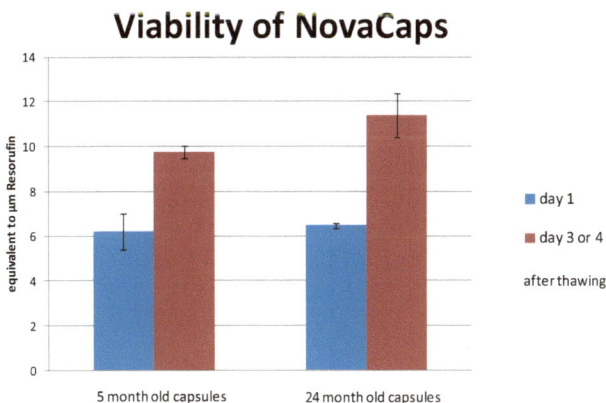

Figure 6: Viability of cells encapsulated in sodium cellulose sulphate after unfreezing. Cell-in-a-Box® capsules frozen at -80⁰C by means of a propriety process were unfrozen after five and twenty-four months and cultivated under normal conditions. Cell viability was equally high after both time periods and cells recover to full metabolic activity (as measured using an enzymatic assay) after three to four days.

high commercial value since cells can be frozen at -80^0C for storage in chest freezers or transport on dry ice or at lower temperatures between -150 and -178^0C which allows storage and/or transport under the gas phase of liquid nitrogen. Both are equally viable using cellulose sulphate. This long-term storage and long-distance transport option makes product validation and distribution possible, which are both necessary for the development of a mass production of a medical product.

4. PROTOCOL FOR THE MANUAL ENCAPSULATION OF CELLS

1) Add 1 ml of sodium cellulose sulphate/NaCl (1-4% SCS*, 0.9% NaCl) solution to your cell pellet and resuspend it by pipetting up and down until the cells are uniformly dispersed. *Caution: Avoid bubble formation.*

2) Attach the filling needle (18G) to the 1 ml syringe (use luer-lock syringe only) and draw up the cell suspension. *Caution: Do not generate any air bubbles.*

3) Replace the filling needle with the droplet needle (34G) taking care that the needle is screwed firmly in place. Eliminate air bubbles within the luer-lock syringe. Discard the first few droplets.

4) Hold the syringe/needle vertically, 2 – 3 cm above the pDADMAC/NaCl (1-4% pDADMAC[1], 0.9% NaCl) bath. *The needle tip must not enter the bath.* Dispense droplets at a moderate speed of 1 - 2 drops per second, maintaining the same drop height. You may move the needle around slightly to prevent droplets from landing on the same spot.

5) Make as many capsules as required but **do not** exceed 1 minute dispensing the droplets. *(Use timer)*

6) Allow the capsules to harden for 5 minutes, starting the count **from the last droplet**, under constant stirring. Adjust the stirrer speed to ensure that the capsules are moving continuously in the bath.

---

[1]Sodium cellulose sulphate (SCS) and pDADMAC concentrations may vary depending on the viscosity of the material.

7) Discard 50ml of the bath solution and add 100 ml of sterile PBS into the beaker.

8) Restart the stirring to wash the capsules for 10 minutes.

9) Discard 100 ml of the bath solution and add 100ml of fresh sterile PBS into the beaker. Wash a second time for 5 minutes.

10) Discard remaining PBS. Leave just a little liquid to cover all the capsules.

11) Rinse 3 times with 30ml PBS, and then another 3 times with 30ml cell culture media.

12) Carefully place your capsules into an appropriate cell culture vessel and adjust the amount of cell culture medium.

ACKNOWLEDGEMENTS

Thanks to Tan Wee Jin, Pauline Toa and Myo Myint Aung from the Austrianova team for their contribution in the lab and thanks from the Singapore Immunology Network to Wang Xiaojie for technical help and Benjamin Toh and Jo Eyles for useful discussions.

CONFLICT OF INTEREST

The author(s) confirm that this chapter content has no conflict of interest.

REFERENCES

[1]   Lim F, Sun AM. Microencapsulated islets as bioartificial endocrine pancreas. Science 1980; 210(4472): 908-10
[2]   Lohr M, Muller P, Karle P, Stange J, Mitzner S, Jesnowski R, *et al.* Targeted chemotherapy by intratumour injection of encapsulated cells engineered to produce CYP2B1, an ifosfamide activating cytochrome P450. Gene Ther 1998; 5(8): 1070-8.
[3]   Dautzenberg H, Schuldt U, Grasnick G, Karle P, Muller P, Lohr M, *et al.* Development of cellulose sulfate-based polyelectrolyte complex microcapsules for medical applications. Ann N Y Acad Sci 1999; 875: 46-63.

[4]   Salmons B, Hauser, O, Günzburg, WH, Tabotta, W. GMP Production of an Encapsulated Cell Therapy Product: Issues and Considerations. BioProcessing Journal 2007; 6(2): 37-44.

[5]   Löhr M KJ, Hoffmeyer A, Freund M, Hain J, Holle A, Knöfel WT, Liebe S, Nizze H, Renner M, Saller R, Müller P, Wagner T, Hauenstein K, Salmons B, and Günzburg WH. Safety, feasibility and clinical benefit of localized chemotherapy using microencapsulated cells for inoperable pancreatic carcinoma in a phase I/II trial. Cancer Ther 2003; 1: 121-31. Epub June 2003.

[6]   Lohr M, Hoffmeyer A, Kroger J, Freund M, Hain J, Holle A, *et al.* Microencapsulated cell-mediated treatment of inoperable pancreatic carcinoma. Lancet 2001; 357(9268): 1591-2.

[7]   Sarmiento M, Glasebrook AL, Fitch FW. IgG or IgM monoclonal antibodies reactive with different determinants on the molecular complex bearing Lyt 2 antigen block T cell-mediated cytolysis in the absence of complement. Journal of Immunol 1980; 125(6): 2665-72. Epub 1980/12/01.

[8]   Kruisbeek AM. *In Vivo* Depletion of CD4- and CD8-Specific T Cells. Current Protocols in Immunology: John Wiley & Sons, Inc; 2001. p. 4.1.-4.1.5.

[9]   Hathcock KS. T cell depletion by cytotoxic elimination. Current protocols in immunology/edited by John E Coligan [et al]. 2001; Chapter 3:Unit 3 4. Epub 2008/04/25.

[10]   Wilde DB, Marrack P, Kappler J, Dialynas DP, Fitch FW. Evidence implicating L3T4 in class II MHC antigen reactivity; monoclonal antibody GK1.5 (anti-L3T4a) blocks class II MHC antigen-specific proliferation, release of lymphokines, and binding by cloned murine helper T lymphocyte lines. Journal of Immunol 1983; 131(5): 2178-83. Epub 1983/11/01.

[11]   Epstein SL, Stack A, Misplon JA, Lo C-Y, Mostowski H, Bennink J, *et al.* Vaccination with DNA Encoding Internal Proteins of Influenza Virus Does Not Require CD8+ Cytotoxic T Lymphocytes: Either CD4+ or CD8+ T Cells Can Promote Survival and Recovery After Challenge. International Immunol 2000; 12(1): 91-101.

[12]   Lin CC, Chou CW, Shiau AL, Tu CF, Ko TM, Chen YL, *et al.* Therapeutic HER2/Neu DNA vaccine inhibits mouse tumor naturally overexpressing endogenous neu. Molecular therapy : the journal of the American Society of Gene Ther 2004; 10(2): 290-301. Epub 2004/08/06.

[13]   Lengagne R, Graff-Dubois S, Garcette M, Renia L, Kato M, Guillet J-G, *et al.* Distinct Role for CD8 T Cells Toward Cutaneous Tumors and Visceral Metastases. The Journal of Immunol 2008; 180(1): 130-7.

[14]   Atherton SS, Newell CK, Kanter MY, Cousins SW. T cell depletion increases susceptibility to murine cytomegalovirus retinitis. Invest Opthalmol Vis Sci 1992; 33(12): 3353-60. Epub 1992/11/01.

[15]   Newell CK, Martin S, Sendele D, Mercadal CM, Rouse BT. Herpes simplex virus-induced stromal keratitis: role of T-lymphocyte subsets in immunopathology. J Virol 1989; 63(2): 769-75. Epub 1989/02/01.

[16]   Ribas A, Wargo JA, Comin-Anduix B, Sanetti S, Schumacher LY, McLean C, *et al.* Enhanced Tumor Responses to Dendritic Cells in the Absence of CD8-Positive Cells. J Immunol 2004; 172(8): 4762-9.

[17]   Eguchi J, Hiroishi K, Ishii S, Baba T, Matsumura T, Hiraide A, *et al.* Interleukin-4 gene transduced tumor cells promote a potent tumor-specific Th1-type response in cooperation with interferon-alpha transduction. Gene Ther 2005; 12(9): 733-41. Epub 2005/03/18.

[18]   Liu W, Chen X, Evanoff DP, Luo Y. Urothelial antigen-specific CD4+ T cells function as direct effector cells and induce bladder autoimmune inflammation independent of CD8+ T cells. Muc Immunol 2011; 4(4): 428-37.

[19]   Tacchini-Cottier F, Zweifel C, Belkaid Y, Mukankundiye C, Vasei M, Launois P, *et al.* An immunomodulatory function for neutrophils during the induction of a CD4+ Th2 response in BALB/c mice infected with Leishmania major. J Immunol 2000; 165(5): 2628-36. Epub 2000/08/18.

[20]   Lopez AF, Strath M, Sanderson CJ. Differentiation antigens on mouse eosinophils and neutrophils identified by monoclonal antibodies. Brit J Haem 1984; 57(3): 489-94. Epub 1984/07/01.

[21]   de Vries B, Kohl J, Leclercq WK, Wolfs TG, van Bijnen AA, Heeringa P, *et al.* Complement factor C5a mediates renal ischemia-reperfusion injury independent from neutrophils. J Immunol 2003; 170(7): 3883-9. Epub 2003/03/21.

[22]   Ueki I, Abiru N, Kobayashi M, Nakahara M, Ichikawa T, Eguchi K, *et al.* B cell-targeted therapy with anti-CD20 monoclonal antibody in a mouse model of Graves' hyperthyroidism. Clinical Exp Immunol 2011; 163(3): 309-17. Epub 2011/01/18.

[23]   Kim S, Fridlender ZG, Dunn R, Kehry MR, Kapoor V, Blouin A, *et al.* B-cell Depletion Using an Anti-CD20 Antibody Augments Antitumor Immune Responses and Immunotherapy in Nonhematopoetic Murine Tumor Models. J Immuno Ther 2008; 31(5): 446-57.

[24]   Pelegrin M, Marin M, Oates A, Noel D, Saller R, Salmons B, *et al.* Immunotherapy of a viral disease by *in vivo* production of therapeutic monoclonal antibodies. Hum Gene Ther 2000; 11(10): 1407-15.

[25]   Schwartz SD, Hubschman JP, Heilwell G, Franco-Cardenas V, Pan CK, Ostrick RM, *et al.* Embryonic stem cell trials for macular degeneration: a preliminary report. Lancet 2012; 379(9817): 713-20. Epub 2012/01/28.

[26]   Gnecchi M, Zhang Z, Ni A, Dzau VJ. Paracrine mechanisms in adult stem cell signaling and therapy. Cir Res 2008; 103(11): 1204-19. Epub 2008/11/26.

[27]   Ratajczak MZ, Kucia M, Jadczyk T, Greco NJ, Wojakowski W, Tendera M, *et al.* Pivotal role of paracrine effects in stem cell therapies in regenerative medicine: can we translate stem cell-secreted paracrine factors and microvesicles into better therapeutic strategies? Leuk Off J Leuk Soc U S A Leuk Res Fund UK 2012; 26(6): 1166-73. Epub 2011/12/21.

[28]   Gunzburg WH, Salmons B. Stem cell therapies: on track but suffer setback. Current Opp Mol Ther 2009; 11(4): 360-3. Epub 2009/08/04.

[29]   Wang Y, Han ZB, Song YP, Han ZC. Safety of mesenchymal stem cells for clinical application. Stem Cell Int 2012; 2012: 652034. Epub 2012/06/12.

[30]   Fujikawa T, Oh SH, Pi L, Hatch HM, Shupe T, Petersen BE. Teratoma formation leads to failure of treatment for type I diabetes using embryonic stem cell-derived insulin-producing cells. The Am J Path 2005; 166(6): 1781-91. Epub 2005/05/28.

[31]   Zakrzewski JL, Kochman AA, Lu SX, Terwey TH, Kim TD, Hubbard VM, *et al.* Adoptive transfer of T-cell precursors enhances T-cell reconstitution after allogeneic hematopoietic stem cell transplantation. Nature Med 2006; 12(9): 1039-47. Epub 2006/08/29.

[32]   Rosland GV, Svendsen A, Torsvik A, Sobala E, McCormack E, Immervoll H, *et al.* Long-term cultures of bone marrow-derived human mesenchymal stem cells frequently undergo spontaneous malignant transformation. Cancer Res 2009; 69(13): 5331-9. Epub 2009/06/11.

[33]   Mishra PJ, Mishra PJ, Glod JW, Banerjee D. Mesenchymal stem cells: flip side of the coin. Cancer Res 2009; 69(4): 1255-8. Epub 2009/02/12.

[34] Amariglio N, Hirshberg A, Scheithauer BW, Cohen Y, Loewenthal R, Trakhtenbrot L, *et al.* Donor-derived brain tumor following neural stem cell transplantation in an ataxia telangiectasia patient. PLoS Med 2009; 6(2): e1000029. Epub 2009/02/20.

[35] Nagy A, Quaggin SE. Stem cell therapy for the kidney: a cautionary tale. J Am Soc Nephr 2010; 21(7): 1070-2. Epub 2010/06/19.

[36] Thirabanjasak D, Tantiwongse K, Thorner PS. Angiomyeloproliferative lesions following autologous stem cell therapy. J Am Soc Nephr 2010; 21(7): 1218-22. Epub 2010/06/19.

[37] Sarkar D, Spencer JA, Phillips JA, Zhao W, Schafer S, Spelke DP, *et al.* Engineered cell homing. Blood 2011; 118(25): e184-91. Epub 2011/10/29.

[38] Smart N, Riley PR. The stem cell movement. Cir Res 2008; 102(10): 1155-68. Epub 2008/05/24.

Send Orders of Reprints at reprints@benthamscience.net

CHAPTER 4

Inducible Systems for Cell Therapy and Encapsulation Approaches

Viktoria Ortner[1], Cornelius Kaspar[2] and Thomas Czerny[1,*]

[1]University of Applied Sciences, FH Campus Wien, Department for Applied Life Sciences, Helmut-Qualtinger-Gasse 2, A-1030 Vienna, Austria; [2]Department for Pathobiology, Institute of Virology, University of Veterinary Medicine, Veterinärplatz 1, A-1210 Vienna, Austria

Abstract: Encapsulation of heterologous cells allows the production of therapeutic substances selectively in the required tissues of the patient. Thus high local concentrations help to minimise side effects in other parts of the body. Nevertheless, most substances show small therapeutic windows also at their site of action. Furthermore, the timing of the release has to be adjusted to the requirements of the patient and the treatment. Regulation from the outside is therefore necessary to adjust the expression in the transplanted cells.

Keywords: Inducible systems, gene expression, alternating magnetic field, heat shock response, regulated gene expression, heat shock promoter, encapsulation, cell therapy, biological, personalized medicine, temperature increase.

1. INTRODUCTION

In the treatment of diseases, localised high concentrations of drugs can substantially increase the therapeutic effects in the desired tissue compared to a systemic drug supply. At the same time the restriction to a certain area reduces the drug-specific side effects in the remaining body. This is especially evident in cases where toxic effects are used to kill tumor cells, but also for many other applications like tissue regeneration. Ideal for the *de novo* synthesis of therapeutic substances within the patient are therefore gene or cell therapy approaches, which target the proteins to their site of action. This strategy results in high local

---

*[*]Address correspondence to Thomas Czerny:** University of Applied Sciences, FH Campus Wien, Department for Applied Life Sciences, Helmut-Qualtinger-Gasse 2, A-1030 Vienna, Austria, Tel: +43 16066877 3511; E-mail: thomas.czerny@fh-campuswien.ac.at

concentrations of the biologicals directly where they are needed. One example is the release of bone morphogenic protein for bone repair, where a restricted delivery strongly improves the therapeutic effects [1]. Nevertheless, a precise control of drug concentration is necessary to avoid severe side effects like ectopic bone formation. Therefore, even if the therapeutic effect is restricted to small regions, a continuous high level production can cause severe problems [2]. Consequently, a combined strategy of localized and regulated expression is required for advanced applications of biologicals.

One of the basic goals of gene therapy is to provide expression of therapeutic proteins in sufficient amounts and for extended time periods. This aim is intimately connected with safety issues. The cell therapy approach solves the problem by extensive preselection of the producing cells *in vitro*. Encapsulation of these heterologous cells prevents the attack of the host's immune system and thus enables stable expression after transplantation for months [3]. Several approaches using encapsulated cells are currently in the phase of clinical trials, however as discussed above, continuous production of therapeutic proteins only covers a small part of potential applications. As for most pharmaceutical interventions, the dose determines the biological response. Methods for controlled expression are therefore of major importance for second generation applications in cell therapy.

During the last years several inducible gene expression systems have been established (Table **1**), mainly for cell culture purposes. For the application of such systems in the clinics, they have to accomplish some important issues. Firstly, the system must show high inducibility, but low basal expression in the non-activated state. Secondly, the system should not interfere with endogenous pathways and thirdly, it should be controllable over a broad range of intermediate levels allowing a precise adaption to the requirements of the therapy. Closely connected with this is the fast reaction of the system to its stimulus from the outside, in particular for downregulation of expression in cases of overdosage. And fourthly, for long time applications it is important that the system does not evoke an immune response to its components. Today several inducible gene expression systems fulfil the above mentioned criteria at least in part, some are already employed in clinical trials.

Table 1: Induction systems for regulated expression of biological

Induction System	Components	Inducer	Side Effects of Inducer	Kinetics *In Vivo*	References
tet-repressor (TetR)	tet-repressor fusions (TA/rtTA)	doxycycline	intermediate	slow	[4-7]
progesterone receptor (GeneSwitch®)	truncated progesterone receptor-GAL4/ p65	mifepristone (RU486)	strong	slow	[8-9]
ecdysone receptor-human retinoid X receptor (RheoSwitch®)	EcR/RXR linked to GAL4/VP16	muristone A or RSL1	weak	slow	[10-12]
rapamycin induced dimerisation	FKBP linked to ZFHD-1 + FRAP linked to p65	rapamycin derivatives	intermediate	slow	[13-16]
radiation induction	Erg–1 promoter, CArG elements	ionisation radiation, DNA damage	strong	fast	[17-20]
heat shock induction	Hsp72-, Hsp70B- or artificial promoters	heat	weak (localized heat)	fast	[21-26]

2. INDUCIBLE SYSTEMS

2.1. Two Component Inducible Systems

Most of the established inducible systems are regulated *via* small molecules. They induce a transactivator, followed by transcription of the therapeutic gene in a separate expression cassette (second component). Best established among these systems is the tetracycline repressor (TetR) inducible gene expression system, which originates from the *Escherichia coli* tetracycline resistance operon. Fusion of the TetR with transactivation domains allowed the adaption of the system to mammalian cells [4]. Today several advanced versions are available using either activation or repression by the inducers, together with improved sensitivity and reduced background activity [6, 7]. In particular a combination of repressor and activator molecules allows precise control of the on/off state [27].

Activation by small molecules as inducers is also used by other gene expression systems. Among them are the rapamycin- [28], the mammalian steroid receptor-

[29] and the insect steroid receptor [11] based induction systems. These systems can precisely regulate gene expression in cell culture, however during *in vivo* applications the inducer molecules have to reach their target cells by diffusion. Therefore the reaction of the systems is slow, in particular if the inducers are administered orally. For example the TetR system was used to trigger expression of therapeutic substances in gene therapy approaches in mice [30] and in encapsulated cells [31, 32]. The studies showed that regulated expression in these applications is feasible, however due to the slow pharmacokinetics of the inducers a switch of gene expression lasted for several days [31]. All above mentioned inducer molecules are pharmacological modulators and thus can induce unwanted side-effects in the patients. Furthermore, for repeated applications immunogenic responses to the multicomponent systems are to be expected.

2.2. One Component Inducible Systems

In contrast to the two component systems discussed so far, one component systems rely on endogenous signaling pathways which activate a single introduced expression unit. Since no artificial transcription factors have to be produced in the cells, immunogenic responses can be avoided. The best established one component systems use external environmental signals instead of small molecules as inducers. This results in an immediate response of gene expression. Most successful among the one component systems are the heat shock promoters.

The heat shock response is an ancient signaling pathway. Expression of heat shock proteins (HSP) helps the cells to survive in emergency situations. Among other stress factors, hyperthermia is a potent inducer of this pathway. Activated heat shock factor (HSF1) binds to the heat shock elements (HSE) and thus induces the HSP promoters. Consequently these promoters have been applied for induced gene expression. Early attempts used natural heat shock promoters, which are highly inducible upon heat exposure, but due to their high basal activity and complex regulation they show a strong background expression [21, 33]. Several attempts to improve the natural promoters were performed, like reducing promoter length [23, 26, 34, 35] or the introduction of additional HSE [21]. Most radically this approach was carried forward by combining idealised HSE directly with a TATA box [36]. The resulting HSE promoter is strongly inducible and lacks any background expression. Furthermore this completely artificial promoter can be used in a bidirectional manner, allowing the simultaneous expression of two genes. A further advantage of artificial heat shock promoters is the lack of acquired thermotolerance in contrast to natural HSP promoter systems [21, 33].

A drawback of endogenous signaling pathways for inducible expression is an accidental upregulation of the therapeutic protein by internal stimuli. In the case of natural HSP promoters a number of stress factors exist which potentially could induce expression. For artificial promoter constructs this interference is largely reduced. Furthermore HSP promoters get fully activated only at temperatures above 42°C, which rarely are obtained in human tissues. Nevertheless, extensive stress signals could occur in certain situations as for example in tumours and might require an option for increased safety. In this respect the recent successful combination of a small molecule inducible system with an HSP70 promoter has to be mentioned. Only the presence of both stimuli (mifepristone and heat shock treatment) resulted in full activation of the system [37]. In addition to the safety aspects, this combination allowed high induction levels combined with low background expression even for *in vivo* applications.

Heat shock promoters are broadly used for inducible misexpression in model organisms [34, 36], where usually the whole organism is exposed to the elevated temperature. But one advantage of heat as external stimulus is the accurate spatial control available for therapeutic applications. Both focused ultrasound and magnetic nanoparticle mediated heat generation (reviewed in [38]) are already in clinical use for localized hyperthermia treatment of solid tumours [39]. Combinations with natural HSP70 promoters have for example been used for expression of suicide genes in tumours in response to localized heat [22-25].

3. INDUCIBLE SYSTEMS FOR ENCAPSULATION APPROACHES

Recently heat inducible expression could also be combined with encapsulation technology [40]. In this system cells harbouring an artificial HSE-promoter construct were coencapsulated with magnetic nanoparticles. Application of an alternating magnetic field then activates the nanoparticles, resulting in elevated temperatures exclusively within the capsules. The procedure is schematically presented (Fig. **1**).

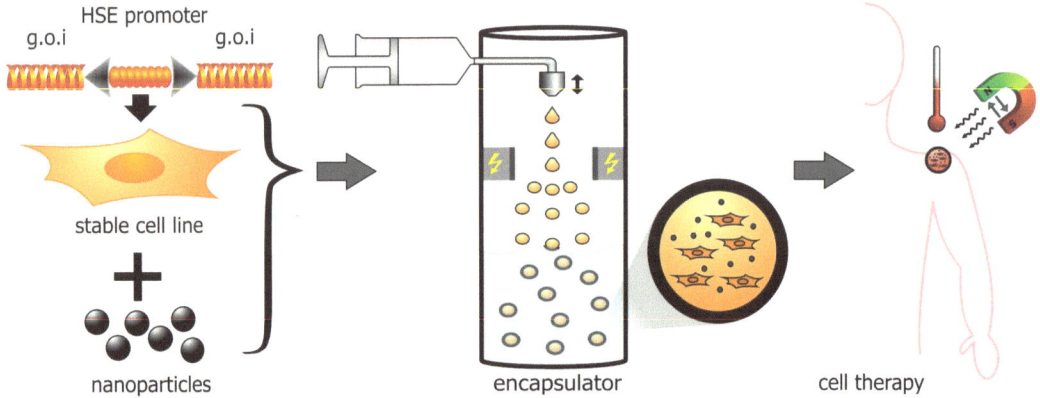

Figure 1: Magnetic field-controlled gene expression in encapsulated cells. Schematic presentation of the heat inducible cells encapsulated together with magnetic nanoparticles, activated in an alternating magnetic field.

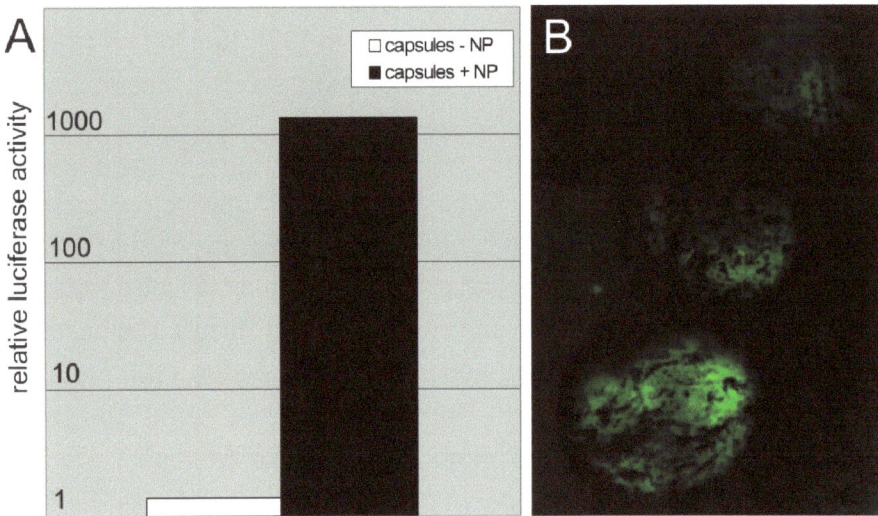

Figure 2: Proof of concept for magnetic field-controlled gene expression in encapsulated cells. A stable cell line containing a heat inducible expression construct driving gfp and luciferase was encapsulated together with (+NP) or without (-NP) magnetic nanoparticles. Activation of the nanoparticles in an alternating magnetic field (60 kHz 27A) activates both luciferase expression (**A**) and gfp expression (**B**) in the capsules.

In a proof of concept experiment (Fig. **2**) it was shown that the system is able to induce reporter gene expression at high levels with low background. Furthermore, the expression could be precisely regulated over three orders of magnitude and reacted to the stimulus within short time. The cells tolerated both the coencapsulated nanoparticles and the heat generated in the capsules. Taken together this recent approach provides full control on the expression in the capsules from the outside, making it a promising candidate for dose-dependent production of therapeutic proteins in patients.

ACKNOWLEDGEMENT

None declared.

CONFLICT OF INTEREST

The author(s) confirm that this chapter content has no conflict of interest.

REFERENCES

[1]   Boden SD. The ABCs of BMPs. Orthop Nurs 2005; 24 (1): 49-52; quiz 3-4.

[2]   Lee RJ, Springer ML, Blanco-Bose WE, *et al.* VEGF gene delivery to myocardium: deleterious effects of unregulated expression. Circulation 2000; 102 (8): 898-901.

[3]   Lohr M, Hoffmeyer A, Kroger J, *et al.* Microencapsulated cell-mediated treatment of inoperable pancreatic carcinoma. Lancet 2001; 357 (9268): 1591-2.

[4]   Gossen M, Bujard H. Tight control of gene expression in mammalian cells by tetracycline-responsive promoters. Proc Natl Acad Sci U S A 1992; 89 (12): 5547-51.

[5]   Gossen M, Freundlieb S, Bender G, *et al.* Transcriptional activation by tetracyclines in mammalian cells. Science 1995; 268 (5218): 1766-9.

[6]   Lamartina S, Roscilli G, Rinaudo CD, *et al.* Stringent control of gene expression *in vivo* by using novel doxycycline-dependent trans-activators. Hum Gene Ther 2002; 13 (2): 199-210.

[7]   Urlinger S, Baron U, Thellmann M, *et al.* Exploring the sequence space for tetracycline-dependent transcriptional activators: novel mutations yield expanded range and sensitivity. Proc Natl Acad Sci U S A 2000; 97 (14): 7963-8.

[8]   Nordstrom JL. The antiprogestin-dependent GeneSwitch system for regulated gene therapy. Steroids 2003; 68 (10-13): 1085-94.

[9]   Taylor JL, Rohatgi P, Spencer HT, *et al.* Characterization of a molecular switch system that regulates gene expression in mammalian cells through a small molecule. BMC Biotechnol 2010; 10: 15.

[10]   Karzenowski D, Potter DW, Padidam M. Inducible control of transgene expression with ecdysone receptor: gene switches with high sensitivity, robust expression, and reduced size. Biotechniques 2005; 39 (2): 191-2, 4, 6 passim.

[11]   Palli SR, Kapitskaya MZ, Kumar MB, *et al.* Improved ecdysone receptor-based inducible gene regulation system. Eur J Biochem 2003; 270 (6): 1308-15.

[12] No D, Yao TP, Evans RM. Ecdysone-inducible gene expression in mammalian cells and transgenic mice. Proc Natl Acad Sci U S A 1996; 93 (8): 3346-51.

[13] Amara JF, Clackson T, Rivera VM, *et al.* A versatile synthetic dimerizer for the regulation of protein-protein interactions. Proc Natl Acad Sci U S A 1997; 94 (20): 10618-23.

[14] Liberles SD, Diver ST, Austin DJ, *et al.* Inducible gene expression and protein translocation using nontoxic ligands identified by a mammalian three-hybrid screen. Proc Natl Acad Sci U S A 1997; 94 (15): 7825-30.

[15] Pollock R, Giel M, Linher K, *et al.* Regulation of endogenous gene expression with a small-molecule dimerizer. Nat Biotechnol 2002; 20 (7): 729-33.

[16] Rivera VM, Clackson T, Natesan S, *et al.* A humanized system for pharmacologic control of gene expression. Nat Med 1996; 2 (9): 1028-32.

[17] Datta R, Rubin E, Sukhatme V, *et al.* Ionizing radiation activates transcription of the EGR1 gene *via* CArG elements. Proc Natl Acad Sci U S A 1992; 89 (21): 10149-53.

[18] Park JO, Lopez CA, Gupta VK, *et al.* Transcriptional control of viral gene therapy by cisplatin. J Clin Invest 2002; 110 (3): 403-10.

[19] Mezhir JJ, Smith KD, Posner MC, *et al.* Ionizing radiation: a genetic switch for cancer therapy. Cancer Gene Ther 2006; 13 (1): 1-6.

[20] Hallahan DE, Mauceri HJ, Seung LP, *et al.* Spatial and temporal control of gene therapy using ionizing radiation. Nat Med 1995; 1 (8): 786-91.

[21] Brade AM, Ngo D, Szmitko P, *et al.* Heat-directed gene targeting of adenoviral vectors to tumor cells. Cancer Gene Ther 2000; 7 (12): 1566-74.

[22] Brade AM, Szmitko P, Ngo D, *et al.* Heat-directed suicide gene therapy for breast cancer. Cancer Gene Ther 2003; 10 (4): 294-301.

[23] Braiden V, Ohtsuru A, Kawashita Y, *et al.* Eradication of breast cancer xenografts by hyperthermic suicide gene therapy under the control of the heat shock protein promoter. Hum Gene Ther 2000; 11 (18): 2453-63.

[24] Guilhon E, Voisin P, de Zwart JA, *et al.* Spatial and temporal control of transgene expression *in vivo* using a heat-sensitive promoter and MRI-guided focused ultrasound. J Gene Med 2003; 5 (4): 333-42.

[25] Huang Q, Hu JK, Lohr F, *et al.* Heat-induced gene expression as a novel targeted cancer gene therapy strategy. Cancer Res 2000; 60 (13): 3435-9.

[26] Vekris A, Maurange C, Moonen C, *et al.* Control of transgene expression using local hyperthermia in combination with a heat-sensitive promoter. J Gene Med 2000; 2 (2): 89-96.

[27] Freundlieb S, Schirra-Muller C, Bujard H. A tetracycline controlled activation/repression system with increased potential for gene transfer into mammalian cells. J Gene Med 1999; 1 (1): 4-12.

[28] Pollock R, Clackson T. Dimerizer-regulated gene expression. Curr Opin Biotechnol 2002; 13 (5): 459-67.

[29] Tsai SY, O'Malley BW, DeMayo FJ, *et al.* A novel RU486 inducible system for the activation and repression of genes. Adv Drug Deliv Rev 1998; 30 (1-3): 23-31.

[30] Furth PA, St Onge L, Boger H, *et al.* Temporal control of gene expression in transgenic mice by a tetracycline-responsive promoter. Proc Natl Acad Sci U S A 1994; 91 (20): 9302-6.

[31] Sommer B, Rinsch C, Payen E, *et al.* Long-term doxycycline-regulated secretion of erythropoietin by encapsulated myoblasts. Mol Ther 2002; 6 (2): 155-61.

[32]   Fluri DA, Kemmer C, Daoud-El Baba M, *et al.* A novel system for trigger-controlled drug release from polymer capsules. J Control Release 2008; 131 (3): 211-9.

[33]   O'Connell-Rodwell CE, Shriver D, Simanovskii DM, *et al.* A genetic reporter of thermal stress defines physiologic zones over a defined temperature range. FASEB J 2004; 18 (2): 264-71.

[34]   Smith RC, Machluf M, Bromley P, *et al.* Spatial and temporal control of transgene expression through ultrasound-mediated induction of the heat shock protein 70B promoter *in vivo*. Hum Gene Ther 2002; 13 (6): 697-706.

[35]   Dreano M, Brochot J, Myers A, *et al.* High-level, heat-regulated synthesis of proteins in eukaryotic cells. Gene 1986; 49 (1): 1-8.

[36]   Bajoghli B, Aghaallaei N, Heimbucher T, *et al.* An artificial promoter construct for heat-inducible misexpression during fish embryogenesis. Dev Biol 2004; 271 (2): 416-30.

[37]   Vilaboa N, Fenna M, Munson J, *et al.* Novel gene switches for targeted and timed expression of proteins of interest. Mol Ther 2005; 12 (2): 290-8.

[38]   Rome C, Couillaud F, Moonen CT. Spatial and temporal control of expression of therapeutic genes using heat shock protein promoters. Methods 2005; 35 (2): 188-98.

[39]   Thiesen B, Jordan A. Clinical applications of magnetic nanoparticles for hyperthermia. Int J Hyperthermia 2008; 24 (6): 467-74.

[40]   Ortner V, Kaspar C, Halter C, *et al.* Magnetic field-controlled gene expression in encapsulated cells. J Control Release 2012; 158 (3): 424-32.

CHAPTER 5

Cell Encapsulation Technology: An Alternative Biotechnological Platform for the Treatment of Central Nervous System Diseases

Tania López-Méndez[1,2], Ainhoa Murua[1,2]†, José L. Pedraz[1,2], Rosa M. Hernández[1,2] and Gorka Orive[1,2]

[1]NanoBioCel Group, Laboratory of Pharmaceutics, University of the Basque Country, School of Pharmacy, Vitoria-Gasteiz, Spain; [2]Networking Biomedical Research Center on Bioengineering, Biomaterials and Nanomedicine, CIBER-BBN, Vitoria-Gasteiz, Spain

Abstract: Cell encapsulation technology is based on the immobilization of cells that secrete active therapeutic agents, in structures made from different biomaterials and surrounded by a semipermeable membrane that protects the cells from the host immune response and the mechanical stress. This technology has proven to be a suitable treatment strategy for different kinds of diseases such as diabetes, heart failure, anemia, cancer or central nervous system (CNS) diseases since promising results have been obtained in numerous works that have been carried out in this field. For this last application, cell encapsulation technology presents exceptional features as it allows direct, continuous and long-lasting release of the desired therapeutic product, next to the affected tissue and without crossing the blood-brain-barrier (BBB). Numerous studies have been carried out using this technology, in different animal models of CNS diseases, in which encouraging results have been obtained. Moreover, the rapid developments achieved in recent years, have allowed the application of these strategies in several advanced clinical trials, reflecting the potential of these techniques. However, there are still some features that must be optimized before cell encapsulation technology can be applied in clinical practice. This chapter will focus on the application of cell encapsulation technology in the treatment of CNS diseases, such as epilepsy, different neurodegenerative disorders- Parkinson, Alzheimer, Amyotrophic lateral sclerosis or Huntington-, pathologies caused by traumas or ischemic processes and brain tumors.

Keywords: Cell encapsulation, cell therapy, biomaterials, central nervous system diseases, neurodegenerative diseases, neurotrophic factor, neuroprotection, neuroregeneration, brain, hollow fiber, alginate, alzheimer's disease, parkinson's disease, huntington's disease, epilepsy, amyotrophic lateral sclerosis, cerebral ischemia, traumatic brain injury, chronic pain, brain tumors.

*Address correspondence to Gorka Orive: NanoBioCel Group, Laboratory of Pharmaceutics, University of the Basque Country, School of Pharmacy, Vitoria-Gasteiz, Spain; Tel: +34 663027696; Fax: +34 945013040; E-mail: gorka.orive@ehu.es
† Deceased.

1. INTRODUCTION

Damage to the central nervous system may be produced by a variety of causes: infection, hypoxic conditions, stroke, trauma of different characteristics or chronic degenerative diseases, among others [1]. All these diseases have in common the fact that, in all of them, a loss of different neuron populations is produced and, thus, serious damage to the individual. Neural regeneration is a phenomenon that does not occur in all types of neurons - neurogenesis has been recently reported in brain areas such as the piriform cortex, corpus callosum and the hypothalamus [2]- and, when it occurs, it is a very slow process, so this type of damage usually is associated to serious consequences.

Today, there are marketed drugs that delay, or at least reduce, the symptoms produced by some of these diseases but there is no treatment available that can completely restore the lost function in a certain area of the brain, caused by neuronal mass death, or to stop the progressive neurodegeneration that can be seen in diseases such as Alzheimer or Parkinson. Advances in understanding the processes that occur in central nervous system diseases are enabling their evaluation from new points of view, which is leading the scientific community to think about new treatment options for neural protection, repair or restoration.

Among the different strategies that are being developed, we find the administration of various therapeutic products such as neurotrophic factors and other growth factors which, by different mechanisms, can protect neuronal function, as it has been demonstrated in Alzheimer, Parkinson, Huntington or epilepsy, among other diseases [5]. Neurotrophic factors are molecules that regulate the differentiation, development and maintenance of neuronal phenotype, synaptogenesis and axon and dendrite development [3] and that, sometimes, can protect neurons from damage and cell death [4]. Moreover, anti-inflammatory molecules have also proven to be effective in reducing neuronal damage because they minimize the gliotic reaction in the brain when trauma occurs, allowing neuronal and axonal growth [1].

Although these strategies are certainly promising, several obstacles must be overcome. One of the most critical problems in the use of such neuroprotective molecules is that most of them cannot cross the blood brain barrier (BBB), so they are inactive when administered systemically (Fig. **1**) [6,7]. Because of this biological barrier, 98% of small molecules and almost 100% of the large ones cannot reach the central nervous system [8], in fact, to cross the BBB in a meaningful way, a molecule must have a high lipid solubility and a molecular weight of less than 400 Da [9]. For this reason, in many cases, it is necessary to administer high doses of drugs systemically to achieve high enough concentrations in the parenchyma [10], causing serious side effects. However, direct administration to the brain, as an alternative to the systemic route, results more aggressive and thus might be careful when thinking about this type of therapeutic strategy.

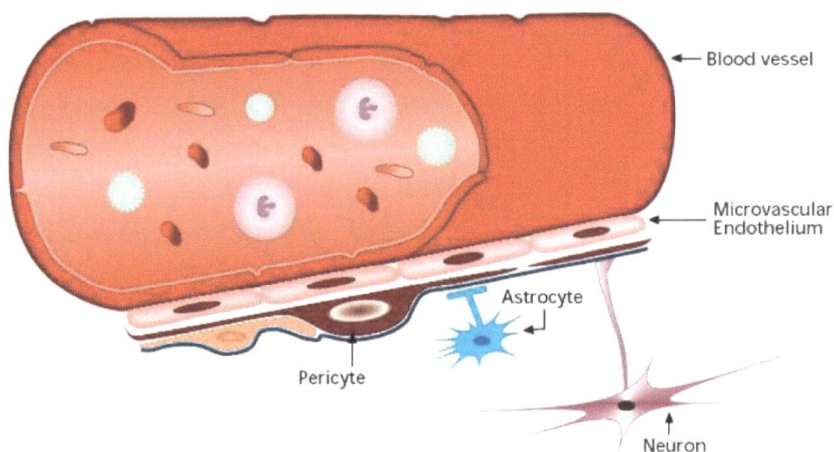

Figure 1: Illustration of the components of the blood-brain barrier, including endothelial cells with tight junctions, pericytes, perivascular macrophages, astrocytic foot processes and drug efflux transporters. Reproduced, with permission, from Ref. [6] © 2011 Bentham Science Publishers Ltd.

Therefore, taking into account that delivering drugs into the brain is certainly one of the most difficult issues to deal with when developing effective therapeutic treatments for diseases of the CNS, in recent years various strategies have been investigated to achieve the protection of the brain against the mechanisms of various neurodegenerative diseases and to repair the neuronal damage associated with traumatic or ischemic conditions.

These strategies have focused on the development of various delivery mechanisms for drugs that prevent degradation of the therapeutic substance before it reaches the selected target and to enhance the drug's ability to cross the BBB, obtaining higher concentrations in the brain at lower doses. Among the most studied mechanisms, we find liposomes [11-13], polymeric nanoparticles [14] (which include nanospheres and nanocapsules), or solid lipid nanoparticles (SLN), dendrimers and micelles [15,16].

Another strategy that is proving to be very interesting in the treatment of CNS diseases is the technology of cell encapsulation. Therapies based on this technology allow direct administration to the CNS, without crossing the BBB, which is especially useful to deliver therapeutics, like neurotrophins [17,18], that cannot be delivered systemically because of significant side-effects or short half life for example. Cell encapsulation also provides a long-sustained release that avoids the need for repeated administrations. Therefore, it presents exceptional features for the direct administration of therapeutic molecules into the brain.

This review will focus on this last therapeutic strategy, cell encapsulation technology, and its most up to date applications in the treatment of CNS diseases.

2. CELL ENCAPSULATION TECHNOLOGY

Cell encapsulation is based on the immobilization of cells that secrete active therapeutic agents in structures made from various biocompatible materials that ultimately surround the cells with a semipermeable membrane [1]. The objective of this membrane is to protect cells from the host immune response and mechanical stress that may occur after capsules are implanted into a particular tissue, while allowing bidirectional diffusion of nutrients, oxygen and cellular waste [19]. Whilst the concept of the capsule is also to localize the cells at the site of implantation and allow the possibility of removal of the cells after the therapy is complete.

Using this technology, we can obtain a sustained, continuous and long-lasting release of the desired therapeutic product synthesized "*de novo*" by the encapsulated cells, which leads to obtain more physiological concentrations while minimizing the risk of toxicity in case of rupture of the device, and also allowing a precise control of the modified entrapped cells in case of significant side effects

[19]. On the other hand, it is important to notice that different release profiles can be obtained by technologically controlling (by means of genetic modification of the entrapped cells) drug or protein release [20] or by modulating the cutoff of the semipermeable membrane. Interestingly, the genome of the host will not be altered, decreasing the risk of tumor formation [21]. An ideal system would be one that achieves an effective concentration of the desired molecule in the target tissue, while minimizing systemic exposure.

This strategy has provided a wide range of promising therapeutic treatments for different kinds of diseases, such as diabetes [22-24], bone and cartilage defects [25-27], cancer [28-30], heart failure [31-33] or anemia [34-36]. Furthermore, to date some clinical trials have been conducted with promising results [37-39].

Although it is clear that this technology could be particularly useful for creating future treatments for central nervous system diseases, there are still some aspects that must be optimized. For example, it is essential to select a cell type which presents a low ability to proliferate once encapsulated (to avoid problems such as capsule breakage [40] or formation of cellular aggregates [41]) and with a constant rate of therapeutic substance release to avoid differences in production between capsules [42-44]. Likewise, the size of the capsule should also adapt to the implantation site. In the case of intravitreal administration or direct implantation into the central nervous system, for example, a smaller capsule size may be more appropriate [45] (Supportive/Supplementary Material).

In addition, for some encapsulation technologies, aspects relating to the capsule biocompatibility and security must be improved before they can be applied in the clinic. Recently, some studies have been published with interesting results about these two issues [46, 47].

2.1. Cell Encapsulation Strategies

Cell encapsulation methods can be classified based on different criteria.

Based on capsule size, there are two types of cell encapsulation: micro- and macro-encapsulation (Fig. **2**). In the method of micro-encapsulation (capsules of about 100-600 μm [5]), cells are embedded within a thin, spherical and semipermeable polymeric layer, while the technique of macro-encapsulation (capsules of a few millimeters or a few centimeters [5]) consists of filling a semipermeable hollow fiber, generally cylindrical, with cells that are normally suspended in extracellular matrix (to improve cell viability and maintain structural support to cells) [1].

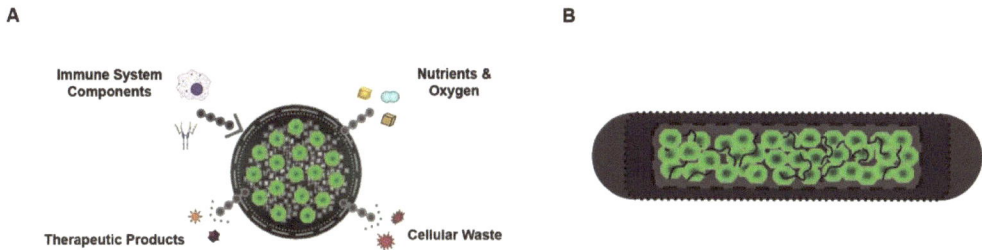

Figure 2: An schematic illustration of the semipermeable membrane allowing the bidirectional diffusion of nutrients, oxygen, therapeutic products and waste while at the same time avoiding the entrance of immune cells and antibodies. (A). Microcapsule. (B) Hollow fiber.

Both bioencapsulation methods have advantages and disadvantages: for micro-encapsulation, the small size of the capsule, its spherical shape and the thin polymer layer surrounding the cells allow an optimal diffusion of molecules through the semipermeable membrane and an appropriate release profile, as well as good cell viability. On the other hand, macro-encapsulation of cells within thicker layers of polymer and larger diameters can increase implant stability [1] and makes it easier to extract the capsule if it is needed [48] but may hinder the diffusion of oxygen and nutrients into the capsules as well as release of waste products, compromising cell viability and the release of therapeutic agents at the same time [1].

In the case of microencapsulation, the materials used vary from polysaccharides to thermoplastics [49]. The polymers used in macro-encapsulation form thicker layers around the cells [1].

Another way of classifying cell encapsulation methods is based on the type of cell used. Based on this criterion, we can find encapsulation of autologous, allogenic or xenogenic cells. There is still controversy of which type of cell is more suitable for encapsulation [50]. Cells for cellular xenotransplants may be obtained more easily but the risk of zoonosis [51, 52], the presence of xenogenic antigens such as galactosyl (Gal) epitopes and the specific functions of xenocells reduce their biosafety and make them more sensitive to immune response [53].

The cell type used for encapsulation can also be classified as primary cells, genetically modified cells or stem cells [19].

2.2. Biomaterials

The use of different biomaterials is beginning to have great importance in the treatment of central nervous system diseases. The materials that are nowadays being developed are allowing and increasing targeted delivery of proteins and drugs into the brain helping, in this way, to repair the damaged neural systems. In addition, using certain biomaterials specific developmental processes and cellular responses such as differentiation, migration and growing processes can be induced. In recent years, these materials are being used also in combination with stem cell therapies due to the fact that they may influence stem cell fate [1].

In cell encapsulation technology, many different materials are used. Among them, alginates are the most common today because they are abundant, readily available and have good gelation properties. As a natural polymer, alginate appears in seaweed and in some bacteria [54].

When working with alginates, there are two properties with which special care should be taken: composition and purity. As for the composition, alginates are a family of unbranched binary copolymers of $1 \rightarrow 4$ linked β-D-mannuronic acid (M) and α-L-guluronic acid (G), of widely varying compositions and sequential structures. It is very important to identify and standardize the differences that may exist in the composition of the different alginates as the composition can vary significantly some properties of alginate gels such as biocompatibility, stability, mechanical strength, biodegradability or permeability. On the other hand, as it is a natural polymer, alginates have great tendency to be contaminated with endotoxins and proteins, which are directly associated with lower biocompatibility. It is therefore an indispensable requirement to carry out an efficient purification process before the use of alginates to make it of a clinical grade [55].

Other natural and synthetic polymers are also under investigation [56] and capsules have been developed for different studies but none have resulted to be as appropriate as alginates. Some of the biomaterials that can be used alternatively to alginate include: poly-ethylene glycol (PEG), chitosan, collagen, hyaluronic acid, dextran, agarose and poly(lactic-*co*-glycolic acid) (PLGA) [19].

To control proliferation and even neuronal differentiation, there is the possibility of modifying the biomaterials with different peptides and proteins to transform the polymers in materials that resemble the extracellular matrix [57]. Examples of such molecules are RGD, IKLLI, IKVAV, LRE, PDSGR and YIGSR [58-60]. The most used is the first one, the RGD (arginine-glycine-aspartic acid), a peptide derived from fibronectin, a protein present in the extracellular matrix [61,62].

The materials used to carry out the immobilization must be totally biocompatible to avoid any inflammatory reaction which can lead to the formation of fibrotic tissue around the capsule, thus hindering diffusion of molecules through the semipermeable membrane [57]. Moreover, if the capsules are implanted in the central nervous system, a serious inflammatory reaction may also cause brain damage.

3. CLINICAL APPLICATIONS OF CELL ENCAPSULATION TECHN-OLOGY: TREATMENT OF CENTRAL NERVOUS SYSTEM (CNS) DISEASES

This chapter focuses on the application of cell encapsulation for the treatment of CNS diseases, such as epilepsy, different neurodegenerative disorders- Parkinson, Alzheimer, Amyotrophic lateral sclerosis or Huntington-, pathologies caused by traumas or ischemic processes and brain tumors. The application of this technology is obtaining promising results in different studies being conducted both *in vitro* and *in vivo*, making it possible that, in recent years, clinical trials have started to be performed in several of these diseases (Table **1**), but much remains to be done before such cell therapies can be carried out routinely in clinical practice.

Table 1: Clinical trials carried out in central nervous system diseases using cell encapsulation technology

Therapeutic Application	Therapeutic Agent	Type of Capsule (or Material)	Results	References
Parkinson´s disease	Spheramine®. hRPE cell implants	Gelatin microcarriers	Phase II. Did not live up to expectations	[90,91]
Huntington´s disease	BHK cells that secrete CNTF	Hollow fiber	2-year study (device changed every 6 months). 6 patients Variability in CNTF levels. No toxicity	[104]
Alzheimer´s disease	NsG0202 implants (EC delivery/NsGene). Encapsulated NGF secreting cells	Hollow fiber	Ongoing Phase I study. Started in 2008 (NCT01163825)	[115]
Amyotrophic lateral sclerosis	CNTF-producing fibroblast encapsulated into polymers with a vitrogen matrix and implanted intrathecally	Hollow fiber	Sustained delivery of CNTF, no toxicity	[122,123]
Traumatic brain injury	Alginate microcapsules containing allogenic mesenchymal cells, transfected to secrete GLP-1. (CellBeads)	Alginate microcapsules	Ongoing Phase I/II study. Started in 2011 (NCT01298830)	[137]
Chronic pain	Chromaffin cell encapsulation into polymers with an alginate matrix and implanted into the subarachnoid space	Hollow fiber	Prolonged cell survival. No significant reduction in pain	[141]

All these diseases are caused by different mechanisms so the strategies used vary between them. However, all of them share some common points, for example, the associated neuronal cell death. Hence, the therapeutic substances released by encapsulated cells will aim at neuro-protection or neuro-regeneration against cellular damage by means of molecules such as neurotrophic factors or growth factors protecting neuronal systems (Table **2**).

Table 2: Preclinical *in vivo* experiments carried out in different animal models of central nervous system diseases, using cell encapsulation technology

PARKINSON´S DISEASE			
Released Molecule	**Material Description**	**Outcome**	**References**
GDNF	GDNF-releasing fibroblasts, bilaterally implanted into the striatum of parkinsonized rats.	Behavioural and morphological improvements.	[71]

	GDNF-releasing fibroblasts, implanted into the striatum of parkinsonized rats.	Sustained delivery and behavioural improvements.	[72]
	Encapsulated GDNF-secreting cells, implanted into the striatum of rats.	Sustained delivery and neuromorphological improvements.	[73]
	GDNF-releasing BHK cells, unilaterally implanted into the striatum of parkinsonized rats.	Sustained release, behavioural improvements and protective and restorative effects on DA neurons.	[74]
	GDNF-releasing BHK cells, unilaterally implanted into the striatum of parkinsonized rats.	Behavioural improvements and neuroprotective effects.	[75]
	GDNF-releasing C_2C_{12} cells, intraventricularly implanted in parkinsonized baboons.	Neurorestorative potential of GDNF and efficacy/safety of encapsulation technology.	[76]
	Neural transplantation + GDNF-releasing polymer-encapsulated cells into the adult rat striatum.	Improved survival, growth and function of fetal dopaminergic grafts.	[87]
	Human embryonic ventral mesencephalic cell suspension transplants + GDNF-releasing C_2C_{12} cells implanted in hemiparkinsonian rats.	Increased fiber outgrowth.	[88]
VEGF	VEGF-releasing BHK cells, unilaterally implanted into the striatum of parkinsonized rats.	Neuroprotective effects of VEGF.	[77]
	VEGF-releasing BHK cells, unilaterally implanted into the striatum of parkinsonized rats.	Neurorescue effects of VEGF.	[78]
	VEGF-releasing BHK cells, implanted into the striatum of parkinsonized rats.	Better results with low-dose administration of VEGF.	[79]
Dopamine	Dopamine-releasing PC12 cells, implanted into the striatum of parkinsonized monkeys.	Sustained release without immunological reaction.	[80]
Neurotrophic factors and dopamine	APA microencapsulated primary porcine RPE cells, implanted into the corpus striatum of parkinsonized rats.	Therapeutic effects on 33% of the rats.	[81]
	Encapsulated bovine chromaffin cells, implanted into the striatum of parkinsonized rats.	Sustained release and morphological improvements.	[82]

Table 2: contd....

NGF	Adrenal chromaffin cells + encapsulated NGF-releasing BHK fibroblasts into the striatum of hemiparkinsonian rats.	High survival rates, sustained release and behavioural improvements.	[83]

HUNTINGTON´S DISEASE			
Released Molecule	**Material Description**	**Outcome**	**References**
Neurotrophic factors	Choroid plexus from neonatal pigs, encapsulated in alginate microcapsules and transplanted into the rat striatum.	An 86% decrease in lesion size in the striatum.	[98]
	Choroid Plexus from adult rats, encapsulated within alginate microcapsules, and transplanted unilaterally into the rat striatum.	Behavioural and morphological improvements.	[99]
	Porcine CP, encapsulated in alginate capsules and transplanted into the caudate and putamen of primates.	Neuroprotective effect.	[100]
CNTF	Encapsulated CNTF-releasing BHK fibroblasts, implanted into the striatum of monkeys.	Neuroprotective effect.	[101]
	Encapsulated CNTF-releasing BHK cells, implanted bilaterally into the striatum of monkeys.	Decrease in the lesion volume and motor and cognitive improvements.	[102]

ALZHEIMER´S DISEASE			
Released Molecule	**Material Description**	**Outcome**	**References**
NGF	Encapsulated NGF-releasing BHK cells, transplanted into fimbria-fornix-lesioned rat brains.	Sustained release and neuroprotective effect.	[105]
	NsG0202 device with an NGF-secreting RPE cell line, implanted in the basal forebrain of Göttingen minipigs.	Sustained release.	[106]
CNTF	Recombinant cells secreting CNTF, encapsulated in alginate polymers and implanted into the right ventricle of mice.	Cognitive improvements.	[107]
GLP-1	Encapsulated GLP-1 releasing MSC, implanted intraventricularly in mice.	Decreased amyloid deposition and anti-inflammatory and neuroprotective properties.	[111]
VEGF	Encapsulated VEGF-secreting cells, implanted into the cerebral cortex of mice.	Increased angiogenesis, decreased presence of Aβ and tau protein and morphological and cognitive improvements.	[112]

	Encapsulated VEGF-secreting cells, implanted into the cerebral cortex of mice.	Increased angiogenesis and cellular proliferation.	[113]

AMYOTROPHIC LATERAL SCLEROSIS

Released Molecule	Material Description	Outcome	References
CNTF	Encapsulated CNTF-releasing BHK cells, implanted in rats.	Neuroprotective effect.	[118]
	Encapsulated CNTF-releasing cells, implanted in mice.	Neuroprotective effect.	[119]
	Encapsulated CNTF-secreting myoblasts, implanted intrathecally in rats.	Neuroprotective effect.	[120]

CEREBRAL STROKE AND/OR ISCHEMIA

Released Molecule	Material Description	Outcome	References
GDNF	Encapsulated GDNF-secreting BHK cells, implanted into the left cerebrum of rats.	Neuroprotective effect.	[127]
	Encapsulated GDNF-releasing BHK cells, implanted into the left brain parenchyma of rats.	Neuroprotective effects and behavioural improvements.	[128]
Neurotrophic factors	Choroid plexus isolated from adult rats, encapsulated within alginate microcapsules and implanted in rats.	Reduction in both motor and neurological abnormalities and decreased volume of striatal infarction.	[129]
	Intracranial transplantation of encapsulated CP into rats.	Improved behavioural performance and decreased volume of infarction.	[130]
VEGF	Encapsulated VEGF-secreting cells, implanted in the striatum of rats.	Reduced volume of the infracted area, angiogenesis and gliogenesis and behavioural improvements.	[131]

TRAUMATIC BRAIN INJURY

Released Molecule	Material Description	Outcome	References
BDNF	Encapsulated BDNF-producing fibroblasts, grafted into the spinal cord of a murine model.	Partial recovery of forelimb usage and axonal growth.	[135]
GLP-1	Encapsulated GLP-1-releasing MSCs, implanted into the right lateral ventricle.	Neuroprotective effects.	[132]

Table 2: contd....

CHRONIC NEUROPATHIC PAIN			
Released Molecule	**Material Description**	**Outcome**	**References**
Neurotrophic factors, catecholamines and opioid peptides.	Encapsulated bovine chromaffin cells, implanted into the rat spinal subarachnoid space.	Pain sensitivity reduction.	[139]
	Encapsulated bovine-derived chromaffin cells, intrathecally implanted in rats.	Sustained release and reduction of mechanical and cold allodynia.	[141]
	Intrathecal implantation of encapsulated HCCs in rats.	Reduction of cold allodynia.	[142]
	Encapsulated PC12 cells, implanted into the lumbar subarachnoid space of rats.	Reduction of cold allodynia.	[143]
BRAIN TUMORS			
Released Molecule	**Material Description**	**Outcome**	**References**
Endostatin	Encapsulated endostatin-releasing cells, implanted into the rat brain.	Inhibition of tumor growth.	[149]
	Encapsulated endostatin-releasing BHK cells, implanted into the rat brain.	Inhibition of tumor growth.	[150]
	Encapsulated endostatin-secreting cells, implanted into the rat brain.	Sustained release and reduction in tumor cell migration and invasion.	[151]
PEX	Encapsulated PEX-releasing MSCs, implanted in mice.	Significant reduction in tumor volume and decrease in blood vessel formation and tumor cell proliferation.	[152]
Anti-EGFR-sTRAIL protein	Encapsulated anti-EGFR-sTRAIL protein releasing CHO-K1 cells, implanted in mice brains.	Sustained release without detectable immunological tissue response.	[155]
EPILEPSY			
Released Molecule	**Material Description**	**Outcome**	**References**
Adenosine	Encapsulated adenosine-releasing BHK fibroblasts, implanted into the lateral ventricle of rats.	Nearly complete suppression from behavioural seizures.	[164]
	Encapsulated adenosine-secreting murine C_2C_{12} myoblasts, implanted in the lateral brain ventricles of rats.	Seizure suppression.	[165]
GDNF	Encapsulated GDNF-releasing cells, implanted into the hippocampus of rats.	Supression of generalized seizures.	[166]

BDNF	Encapsulated BDNF-secreting BHK cells, implanted in the brain of rats.	Amelioration of seizure stage and neuroprotective properties.	[167]

3.1. Parkinson´s Disease

One important neurodegenerative disorder to take into consideration is Parkinson's disease (PD). This disease is characterized by an extensive loss and degeneration of dopaminergic neurons in the substantia nigra pars compacta and their terminals in the striatum [54] with the manifestation of tremor, akinesia, rigidity and disturbances of postural reflexes. The established therapies for Parkinson´s disease are, principally, the L-DOPA drug and surgeries including deep brain stimulation [63].

Since cell encapsulation technologies started to be developed, PD has been one of the major target diseases and different strategies have been tried to reduce the symptomatology and progressive loss of neurons observed in this pathology. Already in the 90's encapsulated cells secreting different molecules for the treatment of this disease were tested in animals [64, 65].

To date numerous studies using cell encapsulation have been carried out, and although results are promising in preclinical stages, there are still several obstacles to overcome in order to bring it closer to a clinical reality. One of the most important issues is that the majority of studies have been conducted in murine models (mainly rats) and therefore there are important differences that must be taken into consideration [66]. For example, in the animal model only dopaminergic neurons are affected whereas in human PD several systems are damaged. On the other hand, the damage that is created in the brains of animals to resemble Parkinson´s injuries in most cases is produced with a chemical substance, such as 6-hydroxydopamine (6-OHDA), that acutely and fast injures dopaminergic neurons, whilst in humans it is a long and progressive process [5].

Nowadays, the glial cell-derived neurotrophic factor (GDNF) is one of the molecules that is most commonly being investigated for the treatment of this disease as it is one of the most potent protective neurotrophic factors for dopaminergic nigral neurons in experimental models of PD [67]. Four clinical trials have already been conducted with GDNF administration in patients with PD with very diverse outcomes. In the first study, GDNF was injected by infusion into the cerebral ventricles without any symptomatic improvement and with reported adverse events, as nausea and depression [68], probably because the protein did not diffuse into the brain parenchyma [69]. In the other three clinical trials, the GDNF protein was infused directly into the striatum. In two of these trials, researchers reported clinical improvements of UPDRS score [70-72], however, the last study failed to demonstrate significant clinical benefits (Thousand Oaks, CA, USA).

While these tests are not very conclusive, experimental studies carried out using the technology of cell encapsulation in different animal models have made it possible to observe that the controlled and sustained delivery obtained with this strategy can greatly improve these results.

However, there are still many unclear points in the use of this molecule. For example, one of the factors that is most commonly seen to affect the outcome of results is the point at which encapsulated cells are administered, with respect to time when the injury occurs. Sajadi *et al.* [73] implanted encapsulated genetically engineered fibroblasts to over-express GDNF in rats, a week after the brain damage was caused and there was no significant increase in the number of neurons tyrosine hydroxylase positive (TH+), although the rats in the treated group got better results in the behavioural test, compared with the controls. Similar results were obtained by Grandoso *et al.*, in another study, when the capsules were implanted four weeks after injury [74]. However, in another experiment carried out by Date *et al.* [75], having implanted the capsules two weeks after the injury, an increased number of TH+ neurons could be seen. Because of this variability in the effect of the capsules administered, other studies have analyzed the results specifically relating to the time of administration [76, 77]. In both cases the best results were obtained when the capsules were administered prior to the lesion, which suggests a protective effect (best results in the test of behaviour and increased number of TH+). On the other hand, if capsules were administered after injury, better results were obtained if the administration was carried out within two weeks of the injury than if it occurred at four weeks.

Although most studies have been conducted in rats, Kishima *et al.* evaluated the technology of cell encapsulation using a monkey model of PD. In this case, capsules were implanted in the ventricle and were replaced at different times. GDNF improved to some extent some motor properties of the primates, but did not increase the number of TH+ neurons [78]. The authors blamed in part to the fact that several of the implanted capsules were no longer producing the therapeutic substance when they were replaced.

Another growth factor that has been proposed for the treatment of Parkinson is the vascular endothelial growth factor (VEGF). In studies in which the effects of VEGF released from encapsulated cells in the brain were analyzed, the following results were obtained: VEGF had mainly a neuroprotective effect because, as previously observed with GDNF, the best results were obtained when the administration was prior to the lesion [79] and results tended to be worse if the administration was performed later in time after the damage. However, in all studies, significant differences were obtained, compared to the control groups [80]. Furthermore, it has been observed that too high doses of VEGF have lower neuroprotective potential and greatly increase the risk of edema [81].

Other research groups have tried to encapsulate pheochromocytoma cells (PC12 cells) for the treatment of this disease. In a study that lasted twelve months [82], capsules containing dopamine-secreting PC12 cells were implanted into monkey models of PD. Results showed some motor improvements.

Another strategy of cell encapsulation used for the treatment of PD was that of Zhang *et al.* [83]. In this case, epithelial cells from the porcine retina with ability to secrete various substances such as dopamine, GDNF and brain-derived neurotrophic factor (BDNF), among others, were encapsulated. In this work, significant differences were only seen in the decreased number of rotations, compared with the control group, in three of the six treated rats. Also chromaffin cells known for their natural capability to produce neurotrophic factors and dopamine have been used in some experiments carried out in rats when encapsulated in hollow fibers [84,85]. These implants were effective in increasing the duration of the effect of systemically administered L-DOPA but only for a few weeks.

Finally, strategies which combine the administration of different cell types producing neurotrophic factors from capsules have also been developed with the aim of increasing the survival of the administered cells. As PD is neurodegenerative, the administration of different cell lines [86] has been tested in order to regenerate or restore the affected area. However, these cells present low survival rates [66] and the apoptosis processes start early [87], possibly due to a lack of neurotrophic factors [88]. Therefore, the co-administration of these cells with other encapsulated cells producing neurotrophic factors may be a viable alternative. Thus, in a study in which chromaffin cells were implanted in the striatum of a rat model of PD carried out by Date *et al.* [85], the presence of encapsulated cells producing nerve growth factor (NGF) managed to increase the survival of chromaffin cells that, when administered alone, produced no significant differences in the test of behaviour. In two other studies, encapsulated GDNF-secreting cells were used to enhance survival of ventral midbrain fetal cells [89] and ventral midbrain embryonic cells [90], in a rat model of PD.

In conclusion, although these early preclinical studies are promising, much work needs to be done still and many questions to be clarified. For example, the most appropriate location for administration of the capsules, the duration of the experiments (12 months the longest study) or the major differences between animal models and humans [5]. Therefore, it has not been possible to start any clinical trial involving cell encapsulation for the treatment of PD. However, a few years ago, a Phase II clinical trial was started in which cells of pigmented epithelium from human retina that produced levodopa and dopamine [91] attached to gelatin microcarriers were implanted in the back of the putamen of patients. Unfortunately, the clinical trial was halted due to the high rate of adverse effects noted [92].

3.2. Huntington´s Disease

Huntington's disease (HD) is an autosomal dominant disorder that usually begins in midlife, resulting from an inherited mutation at the IT15 locus of chromosome 4 [93]. HD is characterized by an intractable course of progressive motor abnormalities and mental deterioration caused by the death of gabaergic neurons in the striatum that invariably results in death of the patient [94]. There are no effective treatments to stop or slow the neurodegeneration that occurs in HD. Some medications reduce the associated symptoms but there is nothing to increase patient survival [95]. If therapies can be devised that preserve the structural and functional integrity of the striatum, they could potently prevent the onset and progression of functional decline in HD patients [96].

As for the case of PD, most of the studies related to cell encapsulation for HD have assessed different neuroprotective therapies. This means that these treatments should be applied before the disease has developed. As an autosomal dominant pathology, the early diagnosis is possible, so such treatments could yield considerable benefits [93].

In the case of HD, the animal models utilized to date for pre-clinical studies, like in PD, are prepared with a toxin that causes rapid and aggressive neuronal damage. In this case, the toxin is quinolinic acid. Although this model provides a useful initial assessment of the ability of a given approach to mitigate the loss of striatal neurons, it does not faithfully recapitulate the slowing degenerative nature or the genetic component of the disease. This is an important limitation to note [97].

A good source of transplantable cells is the choroid plexus (CP). Today, it is well defined that the role these cells play in the production and maintenance of extracellular fluid in the brain is by modulating the chemical exchange between cerebrospinal fluid and brain parenchyma, maintaining the chemical and immunological status of the brain, detoxifying the brain, secreting different polypeptides and participating in repair processes that occur after a trauma [97]. However, lately, the fact that the choroid plexus secretes neurotrophic factors with therapeutic potential has begun to be valued [98]. Furthermore, the time choroid plexus remains in culture does not change its neuroprotective capability [99], a very interesting biological feature when considering its development as a medical tool.

In recent years, the neuroprotective effect of the choroid plexus has been studied in rat [100,101] and monkey models of HD. In the case of rats, several experiments have already been made. In a study carried out by Borlogan *et al.*

[100], the animals were treated with choroid plexus of piglets encapsulated in alginate and transplanted into the striatum. Although the behaviour test showed no significant differences from control groups, lesion size induced by quinolinic acid in the striatum decreased by 86% in the treated group. In another study, CP was isolated from adult rats, encapsulated within alginate microcapsules, and transplanted unilaterally into the rat striatum. Three days later, unilateral injections of quinolinic acid (QA; 225 nmol) were made into the ipsilateral striatum. Rats receiving CP transplants were significantly less impaired on the placement test and Nissl-stained sections demonstrated that CP transplants significantly reduced the volume of the striatal lesion produced by QA [101].

In a study carried out in monkeys by Emerich *et al.* [102], cynomolgus primates received stereotaxic transplants of either empty capsules or porcine CP-loaded capsules directly into the caudate and putamen. One week later, they received unilateral injections of QA. Researchers reported that QA administration produced a large lesion in both the caudate and putamen in monkeys receiving implants of empty microcapsules. In contrast, the size of the lesion was significantly reduced (5-fold relative to control implanted monkeys) in animals with identical QA lesion but receiving implants of encapsulated CP. Hence, it seems that implants of alginate-encapsulated porcine CP can prevent the degeneration of striatal neurons typically occurring after QA intra-striatal injections (Fig. **3**).

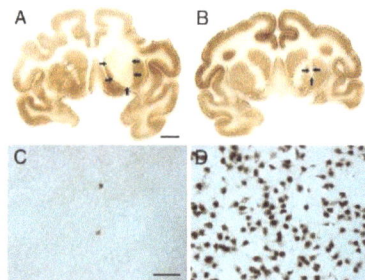

Figure 3: Low- (A, B) and high-power photomicrographs through the striatum of NeuN immunostained sections from (A, C) QA lesion plus empty capsule implants and (B, D) QA plus CP implants in monkeys. Note a large degenerative area seen in both caudate and putamen nuclei in QA lesion side (A, arrows). (B) In contrast, the lesion size was significantly diminished in the CP implanted striatum (arrows). At higher magnification, there were almost no NeuN-ir neurons observed in the QA lesion area. (D) Numerous healthy appearing NeuN-ir neurons were seen in the CP transplanted striatum. Scale bar in panel A represents 0.5 cm in panels B and C and represents 30 μm in panel D. Reproduced, with permission, from Ref. [101] © 2006 Elsevier.

In addition to primary cells, genetically modified cells have also been used to secrete ciliary neurotrophic factor (CNTF) for the treatment of HD. In a study conducted in monkeys by Emerich *et al.* [103], capsules were implanted with baby hamster kidney (BHK) fibroblasts that had been genetically modified to secrete human CNTF and, a week later, QA was administered. This study demonstrated the neuroprotective potential of CNTF on diverse striatal populations, such as cholinergic and gabaergic neurons. In another experiment performed by Mittoux *et al.*, also conducted in monkeys, the toxin was administered weekly for five months during the study and the implantation of the capsules was performed two months after starting the administration of the toxin [104]. Results showed that in the treated group, lesion volume decreased while motor and cognitive functions were improved.

Relying on the promising results obtained in preclinical research, one clinical trial has been conducted evaluating the benefits of encapsulated cells delivering CNTF for the treatment of HD [105]. In this study, developed by Bloch *et al.*, which lasted two years, hollow fibers were implanted in the ventricle of six patients and were replaced every six months. Although no clinical benefits were observed in treated patients, electrophysiological changes were detected in three out of six patients. There are different causes that can justify these modest results. On the one hand, it was shown that cell survival was not very high and moreover many of the encapsulated cells did not produce detectable amounts of CNTF, so the production between different capsules varied much during the study. Furthermore, it is likely that the dose administered was not enough because only one macro-capsule was implanted, whilst, in monkeys it had been necessary to administer four to achieve good results [104]. Finally, in this study the ventricle was chosen as the site for implantation of the capsules, although it had been shown previously that CNTF shows greater effectiveness when administered in the parenchyma [106]. However, a very important and positive fact to take into account is that no adverse effects were detected, so it can be said that this route of administration may be safe and well tolerated.

3.3. Alzheimer's Disease

Alzheimer's disease (AD) is a progressive neurodegenerative disorder associated with age, characterized by memory loss and severe cognitive decline. The neuropathological hallmarks of AD include the accumulation of amyloid beta peptide (Abeta) in both the parenchyma and the cerebral vasculature.

In recent years, several preclinical studies have been published for the treatment of this pathology, using cell encapsulation technology.

In one of these studies, significant protection of cholinergic neurons was obtained by administration of NGF-producing fibroblasts encapsulated in an immune-isolating polymeric device and implanted into the lateral ventricle of rats injured in the fimbri-fornix [107].

In another experiment carried out by Fjord-Larsen *et al.*, a new device of encapsulated cells capable of locally releasing NGF, called NsG0202 or EC bio-delivery, was used. This system, developed by the company NsGene for the implantation of encapsulated cells in the CNS, is similar to a hollow fiber and it is divided into two parts: the lower compartment contains cells surrounded by a semipermeable membrane and measures approximately 1.5 cm in length, while the upper part consists of a catheter which allows removing the entire device from the patient's brain if necessary. This clinical device houses an NGF-secreting cell line (NGC-0295), which is derived from a human retinal pigment epithelial (RPE) cell line, stably genetically modified to secrete NGF. NsG0202 devices were implanted in the basal forebrain of Göttingen minipigs and the function and retrievability were evaluated after 7 weeks, 6 and 12 months. Increased NGF levels were detected in tissue surrounding the devices and the implants were well tolerated but no significant improvements were observed in the treated group [108].

CNTF has also been tested for the treatment of this pathology. In a mouse model of AD, myoblasts transduced to secrete CNTF and encapsulated in alginate microcapsules were implanted intra-cerebroventricularly into mice expressing the mutant amyloid precursor protein, or mice injected with amyloid beta. There were significant improvements in cognitive function [109]. Klinge *et al.,* evaluated the effects of encapsulated mesenchymal stem cells (MSC) derived from human bone marrow, native or transfected to overexpress glucagon-like peptide-1 (GLP-1) in the accumulation of Abeta in a double transgenic murine AD model. This peptide was previously associated with a decrease in amyloid deposition when it was administered by intra-ventricular infusion in normal mice [110,111] and has been observed to protect neurons from Abeta-induced toxicity *in vitro* [112]. In this case, researchers concluded that encapsulated native hMSCs posses anti-inflammatory and neuroprotective properties, which seem to be enhanced by genetic engineering of the cells to secrete GLP-1 [113].

Furthermore, based on the hypothesis that the pathology is vascular, few studies have been performed in which encapsulated cells secreting VEGF (a physiological regulator of angiogenesis and BBB integrity) have been implanted in a murine transgenic model of AD [114,116].

In one of these studies carried out by Spuch *et al.*, the aim was to increase angiogenesis in the brain and, in this way, to enhance the removal of Aß plaques. Results showed increased angiogenesis, decreased presence of Aß and Tau protein, and less apoptosis and cognitive deficits in treated mice (Fig. **4**) [114].

In a recent paper by the same research group, VEGF release from encapsulated cells implanted in a mouse model of AD resulted in an enhanced cellular proliferation in the hippocampal dentate gyrus and in a reduction of the expression and activity of the acetylcholinesterase enzyme, a similar pattern as first-line medications for the treatment of AD [115].

Probably one of the clearest signs that proves this technology is promising also for the treatment of AD is the fact that, since 2010, the first Phase I clinical trial is being conducted, in which encapsulated cells secreting NGF are being used [116]. In this trial, the EC biodelivery system is being tried (Fig. **5**) [117,118]. This system can be removed without difficulty and without risk for the patient, making the application of this technology safer. The data from this trial is not yet published but the devices are reported to be well tolerated and it seems likely that the efficacy will be good.

3.4. Amyotrophic Lateral Sclerosis

Amyotrophic lateral sclerosis (ALS) is a progressive neurodegenerative disease with most affected patients dying after 2 to 3 years.

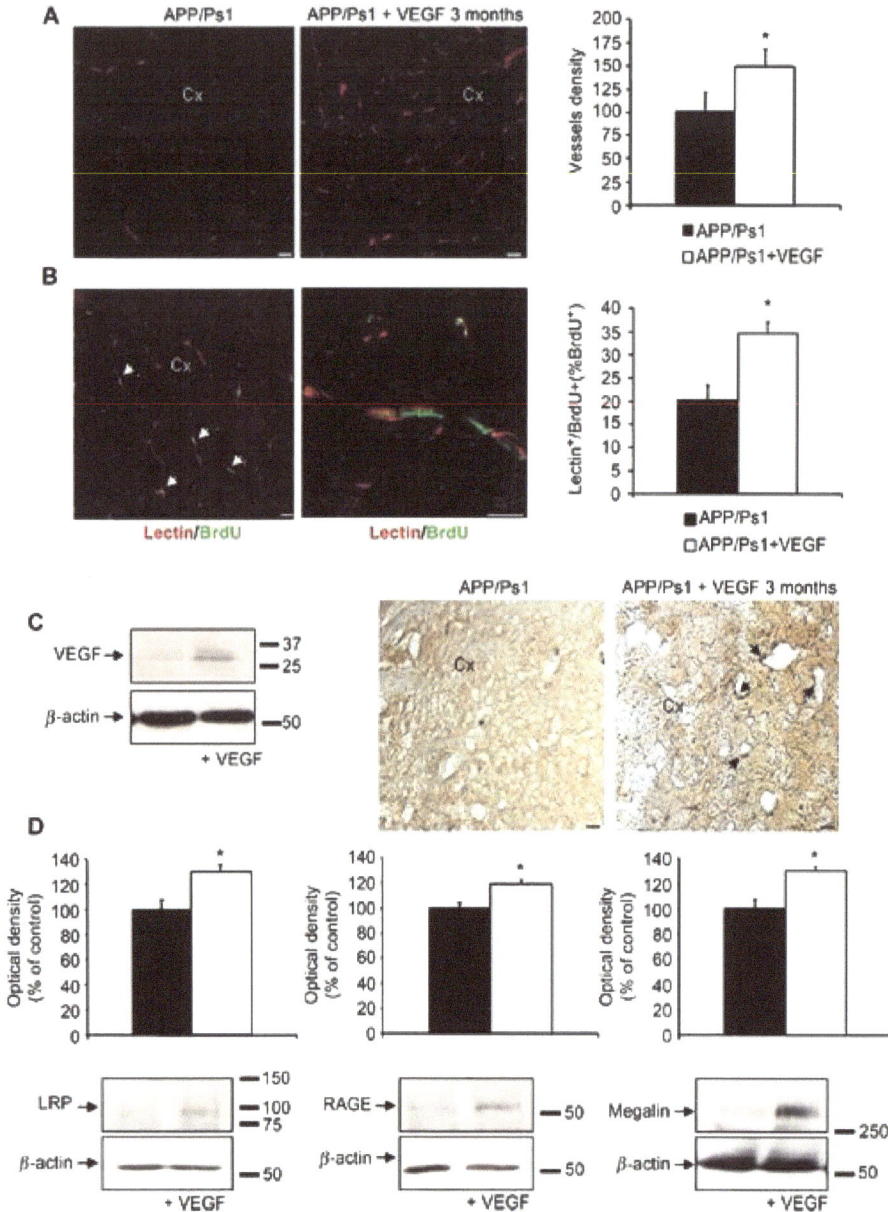

Figure 4: Brain angiogenesis in APP/Ps1 mice after implantation of VEGF microcapsules. (**A**) After three months, implantation of VEGF microcapsules onto the cerebral cortex (Cx) elicits a significant increase in brain APP/Ps1 mice vascularization. Vessels were identified with tomato lectin (red) and the percentage of brain surface covered with vessels was estimated. The histograms indicate vessel density in the cerebral cortex. (**B**) After three months, implantation of VEGF microcapsules induces proliferation of endothelial cells in the cerebral cortex (Cx) from APP/Ps1 mice. Immunofluorescence of newly-formed brain vessels (white arrows) with BrdUrd+

nuclei (green) co-labeled with tomato lectin in the cytoplasm (red). Scale bars = 20 µm. The histograms indicate that the number of double-labeled BrdUrd+/lectin+ cells significantly increased in VEGF microcapsule-treated APP/Ps1 mice. (C) Human VEGF expression was detected in cerebral cortex from APP/Ps1 mice treated with VEGF microcapsule implantation. A representative VEGF blot is shown. Microphotographs of VEGF-stained show VEGF expression in vessels from VEGF microcapsule-implanted APP/Ps1 mice. Re-blotting with b-actin shows an equal protein load in anes (n = 7-8 per group). (D) Implantation of VEGF microcapsules increases expression of LRP, RAGE, and megalin in the cerebral cortex of VEGF microcapsules-treated mice. Representative western blots and densitometry histograms are shown. (Data are expressed as mean ± SEM, *p < 0.05 *vs.* non-transfected cell microcapsules-treated APP/Ps1 mice, n = 7-8 per group). Reproduced, with permission, from Ref. [113] © 2010 Elsevier.

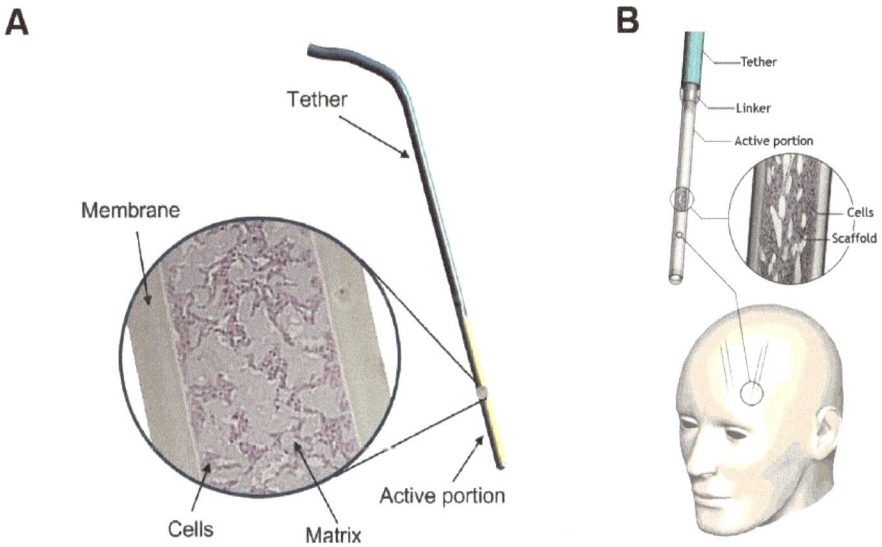

Figure 5: (A). The ECB technology consists of a catheter-like device, less than 1 mm in diameter, suitable for stereotactic implantation in the striatum. The approximately 1.5-cm-long active portion comprises a perm-selective hollow-fiber membrane, which allows for the inward diffusion of nutrients from the surrounding brain and the outward diffusion of GDNF. The long-term survival of the genetically modified human cell line is optimized by the attachment to an artificial matrix. The membrane forms an immunoisolatory barrier which prevents rejection of the allogeneic cell line. In addition, the attachment to a flexible tether allows for the implantation, positioning, and retrieval of the device and the encapsulated genetically modified cells. **(B).** EC Biodelivery™ concept. Reproduced, with permission, from Refs. [116,117] © 2008 Elsevier and http://nsgene.dk/NsGene-416.aspx.

The term "Amyotrophic lateral sclerosis" is used to describe two different but related conditions. The first refers to several adult-onset conditions characterized by progressive degeneration of motor neurons and, the second, to one specific form of motor neuron disease in which both upper and lower motor neurons are affected. The damage in lower motor neurons produces muscle atrophy, weakness and fasciculation and in upper motor neurons overactive tendon reflexes, Hoffmann signs, clonus and Babinki signs. In patients with typical ALS, usually the first symptoms are weakness that starts in hands or legs and includes slurred speech and/or dysphagia. On examination there are almost always lower motor neuron signs together with upper motor neuron signs. If one patient only manifests upper motor neuron signs, this syndrome is considered a variant of ALS, named as primary lateral sclerosis, because at autopsy, there are likely to be abnormalities in both upper and lower motor neurons. Together, the syndromes account for only 10% of all cases of adult-onset motor neuron disease [119].

Studies for ALS have also been performed using genetically modified cells to obtain a sustained release of neurotrophic factors in specific brain areas. In a study carried out by Tan *et al.* [120], BHK cells stably transfected with a chimeric plasmid construct containing the gene for human or mouse CNTF were encapsulated in polymer fibers. Systemic delivery of human and mouse CNTF from encapsulated cells was observed to rescue 26 and 27% more facial motor neurons, respectively, as compared to capsules containing parent BHK cells 1 week post-axotomy in neonatal rats. In a murine model of motor neuropathy, using similar implants, a significant decrease was observed in the motor neuron loss and the survival time was increased by 40% [121]. In addition, macro-encapsulated myoblasts transfected to secrete CNTF have been tested *in vivo* by implanting them intrathecally in rats for 3 months [122]. These implants showed to provide some rescue effect on axotomy-induced neuronal death.

Furthermore, clinical trials have been conducted evaluating the benefits of encapsulated cells delivering CNTF for ALS. In these cases, the implanted cells were safely tolerated without serious adverse events, justifying further clinical evaluation. However, the relatively modest cell survival in these studies will need to be improved [123,124].

In one of these studies in which capsules with BHK fibroblasts modified to produce CNTF were intrathecally implanted in patients with ALS, the immune response was studied for 20 weeks [123]. Authors concluded that there was no significant immune response against the implanted capsules.

Aebischer *et al.*, in a 17-month experiment carried out in six patients, observed that macrocapsules containing CNTF-producing cells implanted intrathecally did not stop the progression of the disease, but on the other hand, no major signs of immune response against the capsules nor side effects were detected [124]. One reason why the results achieved were not as good as expected could be the variability in the levels of CNTF in the CNS detected between the different patients, in addition to the short duration of the study and the small number of patients recruited.

Other biomolecules that have been used for the treatment of ALS are VEGF and GDNF. VEGF has been shown to prevent motor neuron degeneration and prolong survival in superoxide dismutase-1 (SOD-1) mutant rodents; a type of ALS model [125,126]. GDNF, in turn, has demonstrated to increase motor neuron survival, delay disease progression and increase lifespan, when autologous myoblasts or bone marrow-derived MSCs were transduced to secrete GDNF and were implanted intramuscularly into SOD-1 mutant rats and mice prior to disease onset [127,128].

3.5. Cerebral Stroke and/or Ischemia

Nowadays, vascular diseases, such as cerebral stroke, are among the leading causes of morbidity and mortality in developed countries and the ischemia caused by blood flow blockage to the brain or to a particular part of it. Furthermore, they are directly associated with the development of various disabilities. In recent years, advances have been achieved in the treatment of these pathologies, using different strategies, including cell encapsulation.

As in other CNS diseases, for ischemia, studies have been conducted with capsules containing cells producing GDNF. In two studies carried out in newborn rats, significant immune response was not detected around the capsules and the cells were shown to still be viable when the capsules were removed [129]. Furthermore, GDNF also increased the neural survival as it improved performance of rats in various memory and learning tests. Therefore, it could be shown that GDNF has a neuroprotective effect [130].

The choroid plexus (CP) has also been used in ischemia models. In a study by Borlongan *et al.* [131], the CP decreased the lesion size by 25%, while the neurological and motor deficit improved by 40%. In another study carried out by the same researchers, encapsulated and non-encapsulated plexus material was implanted [132]. The immune response detected against the non-encapsulated plexus was much greater than the one seen against encapsulated plexus and this significantly affected its viability. Furthermore, it was demonstrated that the encapsulated plexus significantly reduced the extension of the infarcted brain area and its associated behavioural effects.

Finally, another strategy used was implantation of capsules containing VEGF-secreting cells for 14 days in the striatum of a rat model of cerebral ischemia, performed by Yano *et al.* [133]. In this study, the neuroprotective capability of VEGF was shown as it increased neuronal survival. Implantation of capsules reduced the volume of the brain area affected by ischemia significantly and the results obtained in the behavioural test turned out to be more favorable for treated rats when compared with the control group.

3.6. Traumatic Brain Injury

It is estimated that annually, in the world, 10 million people are affected by traumatic brain injury (TBI) and the highest incidence is among people from 15 to 24 years of age and 75 years and older. TBI is a disorder of major public health significance since it may result in lifelong impairment of an individual´s physical, cognitive, and psychosocial functioning [134]. This pathology results in the disruption of ascending and descending axons that produce a devastating loss of motor and sensory function. Several strategies have been used to provide trophic and anti-apoptotic molecules that can alter the environment of the injured CNS.

Various studies [135,136] have pointed out that primary fibroblasts genetically modified to produce BDNF survived in the injured spinal cord of adult Sprague-Dawley rats rescuing axotomized neurons, promoting regeneration and contributing to recovery of locomotor function. However, immunosuppression was needed to prevent rejection of grafts. As an alternative, cell micro-encapsulation could replace immune suppression by protecting the cells after grafting. In 2005 Tobias *et al.* [137] reported that alginate–poly-L-ornithine microcapsules containing BDNF-producing fibroblast cells grafted into a non-immunosuppressed SCI murine model resulting in partial recovery of forelimb usage in a test of vertical exploration and of hind limb function while crossing a horizontal rope. However, results were similar to those of immune-suppressed animals that had received non-encapsulated cells. The study also showed no evidence of regeneration of rubrospinal axons in mice implanted with encapsulated cells presumably because the amounts of BDNF available from the encapsulated graft were substantially less than those provided by the much larger numbers of cells grafted in the non-encapsulated formulation in the presence of immune-suppression.

Another group conducted a preclinical study testing the effect of alginate-encapsulated native MSCs and alginate-encapsulated GLP-1 transfected MSCs, implanted into the right lateral ventricle, in an experimental traumatic brain injury model [134]. In this study, hippocampal cell loss was reduced, along with an attenuation of cortical neuronal and glial abnormalities, in both of the stem cell-treated groups of animals. The effects were more pronounced in animals treated with GLP-1 secreting hMSCs.

Recently, in 2011, a Phase I/II clinical trial has started in patients with TBI with intra-cerebral hemorrhage (ICH). In this study, alginate microcapsules containing allogenic MSC, transfected to secrete GLP-1 were implanted into the brain tissue cavity after surgical evacuation of the hematoma [138]. Capsules were removed by second surgery after 14 days of treatment. An important fact to note here is that the capsules were not implanted directly into the brain but placed in a small bag of 1.5 x 1.5 cm with pores of about 300 µm, allowing the easy removal after treatment. The first data being obtained from this study showed that there were no serious adverse effects in patients and that cell survival was good (Fig. **6**).

3.7. Chronic Neuropathic Pain

Nowadays, there are different treatments that can help patients suffering from chronic pain to cope with the symptoms of this illness but they are not always completely effective. Some people may live for years with this disease, which in many cases significantly decreases their quality of life.

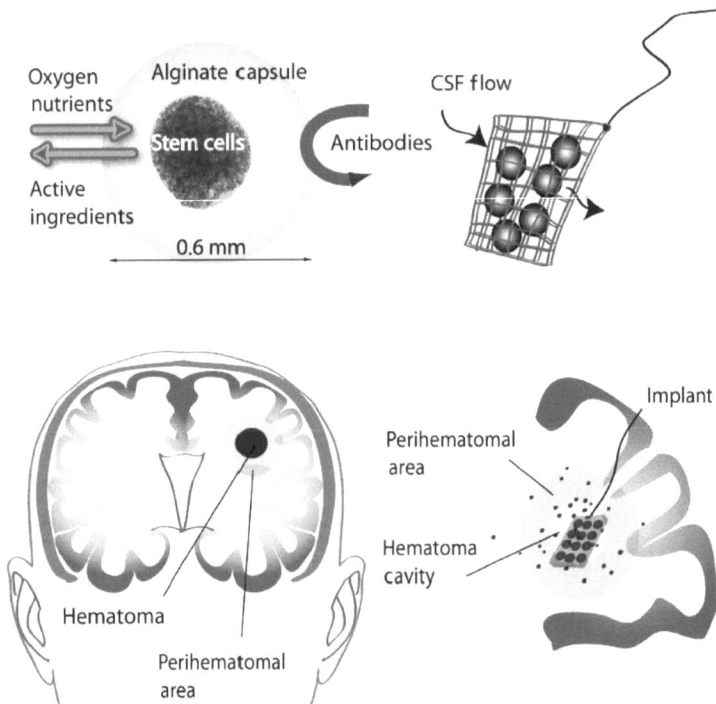

Figure 6: Encapsulated mesenchymal cell biodelivery of GLP-1. Upper left: Human bone marrow-derived, mesenchymal stem cells producing GLP-1 are encapsulated with alginate (capsule diameter 500 to 600 μm, each capsule containing 3200 cells). As the capsules permit the free passage of nutrients, oxygen, and, indeed, smaller molecules, the cells are maintained within the capsules, and can produce and deliver therapeutic peptides to the brain. At the same time, cells transplanted into the brain are protected from the immunological graft-*vs.*-host response. Upper right: The microcapsules are filled into a 1.5 x 1.5 cm-sized bag that is manually sutured from a polypropylene mesh with pores of up to 300 μm. A 5-cm tether for fixation of the implant to the skull surface is applied. CSF can pass through the pores providing the encapsulated cells with nutrients and oxygen. Lower left: The surgical hematoma is evacuated leaving the perihematomal area. Lower right: The mesh bag is implanted into the hematoma cavity, and it is removed 2 weeks after implantation by a second surgery. GLP, glucagon-like peptide; CSF, cerebrospinal fluid. Reproduced, with permission, from Ref. [133] © 2011 LLS SAS.

Cell encapsulation has also been used to try to improve existing treatments for chronic pain. These studies have focused mainly on intrathecal administration of chromaffin cells since such cells constitutively release catecholamines, opioid peptides, and neurotrophic factors [139]. Moreover, chromaffin cells also express nicotinic receptors, which stimulate secretion of these substances when activated by nicotine, a feature that could be utilized *in vivo* to achieve a level of control over release [140].

In one of the first studies carried out by Sagen *et al.*, isolated bovine chromaffin cells were encapsulated and implanted into the rat spinal subarachnoid space. Pain sensitivity was assessed at several intervals up to 3 months following implantation. Results indicated that encapsulated bovine chromaffin cell implants, but not empty control capsules, could repeatedly reduce pain sensitivity for the duration of the study [141].

With this strategy, a Phase I clinical trial was designed in which a human-scale implant containing bovine chromaffin cells was developed, characterized, and implanted in the subarachnoid space of seven patients with severe chronic pain which could not be satisfactorily managed with conventional therapies. The results were quite good as slight improvements were observed in some patients and the survival of the cells inside the capsules was confirmed at the end of the study. It is also important to note that patients did not receive any immunosuppressive treatment despite transplanted capsules contained xenogenic tissue [142].

Another approach to be mentioned was proposed by Jeon *et al.* for the treatment of chronic neuropathic pain [143]. Using a rat model of neuropathic pain, the implantation of encapsulated bovine-derived chromaffin cells resulted in high levels of release of catecholamines and metenkephalin demonstrating the effectiveness of the developed system.

In recent years, more studies have been designed for the treatment of chronic pain with chromaffin cells [144] and PC12 cells [145] in rat models of chronic pain. In the case of chromaffin cells, human chromaffin cells (HCCs) encapsulated within alginate-poly-L-lysine-alginate (APA) microcapsules were intrathecally implanted into rats. Empty capsules were intrathecally implanted as a control. Intrathecal implantation of encapsulated HCCs, significantly reduced cold allodynia as compared to rats receiving empty capsules (P < 0.05). In the second experiment, using PC12 cells, rats with CCI were divided randomly into two groups: the cell-loaded group received microencapsulated PC12 cells and the control group received empty capsules. In this case, microcapsules were implanted into the lumbar subarachnoid space. After implantation, a significant reduction of cold allodynia was observed in the rats of the cell-loaded group at 7, 14, 21, and 28 days compared to the control group (P < 0.05) (Fig. **7**).

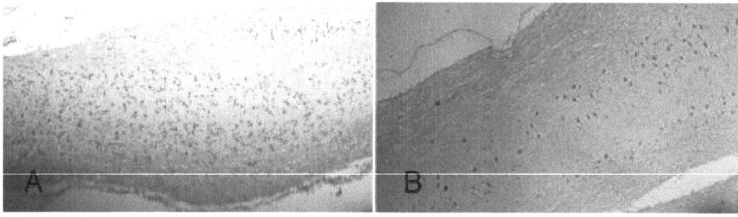

Figure 7: Histological analysis of the spinal space of the rats (A) in the cell-loaded group and (B) in the control group. The samples were removed after 4 weeks of implantation. The tissue sections were stained with hematoxylin and eosin (50 X magnification). Reproduced, with permission, from Ref. [144] © 2010 International Center for Artificial Organs and Transplantation and Wiley Periodicals, Inc.

3.8. Brain Tumors

Another important field of application of cell encapsulation is cancer therapy [146-148]. In the case of patients with tumors in the CNS, they often have low survival rates despite surgery, chemotherapy and/or radiotherapy. Hence, innovative therapies and strategies must be developed to prolong survival of these patients.

Principally there are two strategies for the treatment of different kinds of tumors (Fig. **8**). The first strategy is based on enhancing the immunogenicity of tumor cells, thus allowing systemic immune-mediated tumor cell death. In order to achieve this target several different immune-mediating products, such as antibodies and cytokines, have been assayed.

The production of cytokines, such as interleukins or tumor necrosis factor alpha (TNF-alpha), from encapsulated cells is a potential strategy for the treatment of solid tumors and the results obtained in some studies conducted using this strategy are quite promising as they have shown enhanced immunity whereas risk for tumorigenicity has been decreased [149-152].

Nowadays, there are already some well-established treatments for cancer with monoclonal antibodies, such as herceptin and avastin, which are now on the market. The implantation of antibody producing encapsulated cells, which were first used for the long term *in vivo* production of antibodies at the turn of the

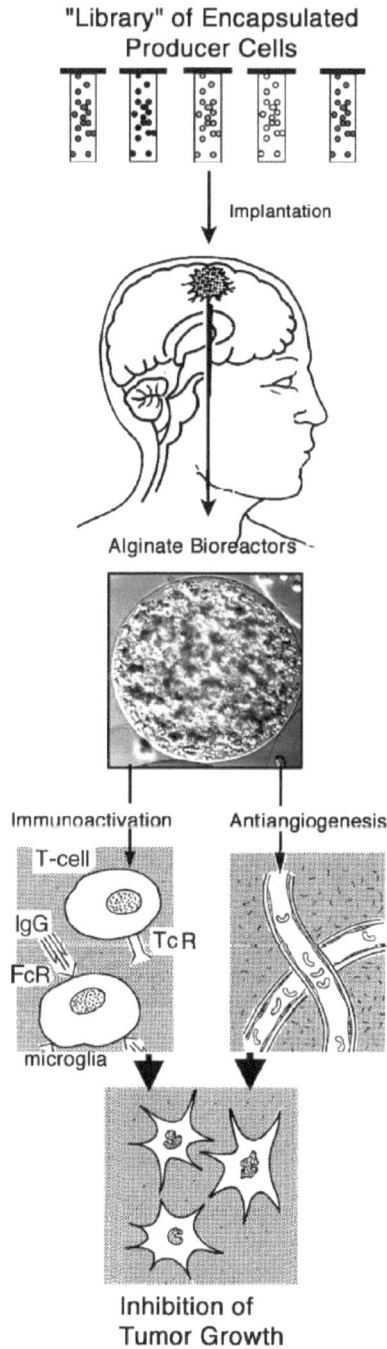

Figure 8: Schematic presentation of the alginate concept used for the treatment of CNS malignancies. Reproduced, with permission, from Ref. [147] © 2001 Oxford Journals.

century [153-156], could improve the therapeutic efficacy of these agents. A continuous antibody production should avoid the peaks and troughs in the amount of circulating antibody that are typically observed with bolus-type delivery. Moreover, new monoclonal antibodies or combinations of antibodies could also be released to enhance the immunogenicity of tumor cells.

Kuijlen *et al.* presented a study in which alginate microcapsules filled with Chinese Hamster Ovary cells (CHO-K1) that were engineered to produce the single chain anti-EGFR-sTRAIL (scFv425:sTRAIL), an antibody fragment which can induce apoptosis, were implanted peri-tumorally. Results showed maintained biological functionality of the released scFv425:sTRAIL protein and that there was no immunological response detectable after intra-cerebral implantation of the alginate capsules in mice brains [157].

The other strategy of interest in the treatment of cancer is angiogenesis inhibition. Tumors are dependent for their growth on the development of new blood vessels that can supply enough oxygen and nutrients for the high degree of growth and differentiation of tumor cells. Therefore, tumor cells usually trigger angiogenesis processes by the release of specific growth factors such as VEGF. Thus, the inhibition of angiogenesis can suppress the growth of tumors [54].

By means of exploiting this second pathway as a method for reducing tumors, in 2001 two independent groups [158,159] treated glioma models of cancer with encapsulated xenogenically derived cell lines genetically modified to secrete endostatin, one of the most potent anti-angiogenic biomolecules that can directly induce apoptosis in tumor cells. Both groups reported that local delivery of endostatin significantly inhibited tumor growth.

Two years later, in 2003, another study [160] was published in which human embryonic kidney cells were transfected with the endostatin gene and encapsulated in calcium cross-linked alginate microcapsules. The capsules, implanted into rat brains showed only a moderate loss in cell viability and extended endostatin release for periods of up to 12 months. The local delivery of endostatin seemed to specifically affect tumor-associated microvessels by reduction of the vessel density, diameter and functionality. Tumor cell migration and invasion was greatly reduced in the endostatin treated animals.

In a recent work, Goren *et al.* [161] encapsulated genetically engineered hMSCs to express hemopexin like protein (PEX), another angiogenesis inhibitor, in alginate–poly-l-lysine (PLL) microcapsules and tested the efficacy of the microencapsulation system in a model of human glioblastoma. They reported a significant reduction in tumor volume (89%), 22 days after the beginning of the therapy, when compared with the control groups. Furthermore, immune-histological studies demonstrated a decrease in blood vessel formation and tumor cell proliferation and an increase in tumor cell apoptosis.

In order to develop more effective therapies, experiments have been conducted combining both anti-tumor strategies, by the simultaneous delivery of cytokines and anti-angiogenic drugs. Cirone *et al.* examined a two pronged strategy by delivering interleukin 2 fusion protein (immunotherapy) and angiostatin (anti-angiogenic therapy) – angiostatin has also been used alone as an antiangiogenic cancer therapy with microencapsulated cells [162,163]- *via* micro-encapsulated cells, to evaluate their potential synergism in tumor suppression. The results suggested improved efficacy over the single treatments [164,165].

Apart from the inhibition of angiogenesis and the strategy of enhancing the immunogenicity of tumor cells, in recent years, other types of cell encapsulation technology applications have also been developed. The use of encapsulated cells over-expressing enzymes that can activate chemotherapeutic agents or prodrugs, for example, is also a promising means to treat tumors [166]. Based on the good results obtained in preclinical studies, NovaCaps®, an encapsulated cell therapy product developed by Austrianova, was tested in a Phase I/II clinical trial which involved the treatment of 14 patients suffering from pancreatic cancer. The results of this trial were very promising since one year survival of the patients was three times higher than that of the currently used gold standard treatment gemcitabine and permission to continue into a Phase III trial was granted by the EMEA. Importantly, Austrianova showed for the first time that it was possible to large scale manufacture, store and ship an encapsulated cell therapy product under current Good Manufacturing Procedure (GMP) conditions. The GMP product NovaCaps® was given product release status by the German authorities for the Phase III trial in 2008. It is interesting to consider that this type of strategy could also be applied for use against brain tumors [167-169].

3.9. Epilepsy

Epilepsy is a common and diverse set of chronic neurological disorders characterized by seizures. These seizures result from abnormal, excessive or hyper-synchronous neuronal activity in the brain. About 50 million people worldwide have epilepsy.

This pathology can be somewhat controlled with medication. However, over 30% of people suffering from this pathology do not have seizure control even whilst they are under treatment [170] and patients whose epilepsy can be successfully treated with anti-epileptic medication usually suffer adverse effects such as dizziness, sedation, impairment of cognitive function and teratogenic effects [171].

Epilepsy is another disease for which cell encapsulation has been used with positive results shown. One of the strategies used is based on the adenosine augmentation therapy [172]. The crucial role of adenosinergic neuro-modulation in the control of seizure activity is well established [173] and it is also known that adenosine is involved in one of several endogenous mechanisms of the brain that is implicated in the finalization of seizures in the return to the interictal state [174]. In a study carried out by Huber *et al.*, [175] where cell encapsulation technology was applied for the paracrine cell-based release of adenosine, BHK fibroblasts were subjected to chemical mutagenesis to obtain a more substantial release of adenosine. These cells were encapsulated in hollow fibers and implanted into the lateral brain ventricle of rats. It was observed that during the first 12 days after transplantation the adenosine releasing devices provided nearly complete suppression from behavioural seizures as well as a reduction of afterdischarges recorded in hippocampal EEGs. However, the principal limitation of this study was the low survival of the implanted cells.

In another similar experiment by Güttinger *et al.,* [176], murine C_2C_{12} myoblasts were engineered to release adenosine, encapsulated in hollow fibers and implanted in the lateral brain ventricles of fully kindled rats. The devices provided seizure suppression in most animals for at least 2 weeks and up to 8 weeks in one animal. Furthermore, in this case, the viability of the cells was better and there were no significant side effects.

Like in other CNS diseases, the employment of neurotrophic factors has demonstrated to be useful in the treatment of epilepsy. In a study carried out by Kanter-schlifke *et al.*, encapsulated cells, which were genetically modified to produce and release GDNF, demonstrated the ability to suppress recurrent generalized seizures when implanted into the hippocampus of kindled rats [177].

Another neurotrophic factor that has been used in the treatment of epilepsy is BDNF, which is a well known molecule with neuroprotective potential. Kuramoto *et al.* observed that rats receiving encapsulated BDNF-secreting cells showed significant amelioration of seizure stage and reduction of the number of abnormal spikes at day 7 after kainic acid administration compared to the control group. They even reported neuro-protective properties of the BDNF release in the brain with enhanced neurogenesis in the treated rats [178].

However, although these studies have retrieved positive results, the benefits of neurotrophins in the context of epilepsy have not been as evident as in other CNS diseases. In animal models, neurotrophins have been shown to have detrimental effects when large doses have been administered, while the continual administration of smaller doses has resulted in being beneficial for reducing the symptoms of epilepsy [177,178]. Therefore, dosage is of critical importance.

4. CONCLUSIONS AND FUTURE DIRECTIONS

Traditionally, therapies for CNS diseases, caused by trauma or neurodegenerative processes, have been very limited and, in general, the few drugs available in the market only provide mild symptomatic relief or little improvement in the clinical situation of patients. Moreover, the benefits obtained with these therapies are usually due to a mere delay in the pathologic mechanisms that ultimately develop, despite treatments.

Cell encapsulation has advanced greatly in recent years, becoming a promising strategy for the treatment of these diseases. These technologies allowing sustained release of biomolecules with therapeutic potential directly to the CNS (thus avoiding the passage through the BBB) are opening many possibilities that extend beyond the symptomatic relief to include neuro-protection and neuro-repair.

The examples presented in this chapter are only part of the studies being carried out worldwide with this technology and the results being obtained *in vitro* and in different animal models are very positive. However, few clinical trials have been conducted to date showing that we are still far from being able to apply the methods of cell encapsulation routinely in clinical practice.

Nowadays, there are still many obstacles to be overcome before this technology can be optimized. Reduction of the diameter of the capsules may be an interesting alternative when the administration must take place in the CNS. Furthermore, cell viability and immune response produced against the capsules are still major problems for some of the more commonly used technologies such as alginate.

Hence, the development of new biomaterials is essential to achieve biocompatible membranes of suitable permeability and strength which can be integrated in brain tissue in an appropriate manner, allowing the release of the therapeutic substance optimally.

However, though much work needs to be done yet, the multidisciplinary collaboration of scientists and clinicians from different areas such as genetics, materials science, chemical engineering, pharmaceutical technology, biology and medicine will make it possible to bring this technology closer to a realistic proposal for clinical application in the upcoming years.

5. PROTOCOL: A STATE-OF-THE-ART STRATEGY TO TREAT CNS DISEASES

5.1. Implantation of Small (100μm) Microcapsules in Reduced Sites. Craniotomy Procedure through Stereotaxy

5.1.1. Elaboration of Microcapsules of Reduced Size (100μm)

Cells are encapsulated into alginate-PLL-alginate (APA) microcapsules using the Flow Focusing System (Ingeniatrics Tecnologías, S.L.), which allows the elaboration of microparticles of reduced size (100 μm) following a brief modification of Lim and Sun's procedure [22]. Ultra pure low-viscosity high guluronic acid alginate (UPLVG) is employed, purchased from FMC Biopolymer, Norway. Poly-L-lysine (PLL hidrobromide Mw 15 000–30 000 Da) is obtained from Sigma Aldrich (St. Louis, MO, USA). Briefly, cells are harvested from monolayer cultures using trypsin-EDTA (Invitrogen), filtered through a 40 μm pore mesh and resuspended in 1.5% sodium alginate at a density of 10×10^6 cells/mL. The resulted suspension is extruded using a sterile syringe through a 0.24 mm diameter nozzle tip (orifice diameter) at a flow rate of 2 mL/h using a peristaltic pump, and focused with sterile air at 90 to 120 mbar pressure. Alginate drops are collected in a 55mM $CaCl_2$ solution and maintained stirring in a shaker for 15min once the process is finished in order to ensure the complete jellification of all the microparticles. Subsequently, the beads are suspended in 0.05% PLL solution for 5 min, washed twice with 10 mL of mannitol 1% and coated again with another layer of 0.1% alginate for 5 min. Finally, microcapsules are cultured in complete medium. The whole process is carried out at room temperature and under aseptic conditions (Fig. **9**).

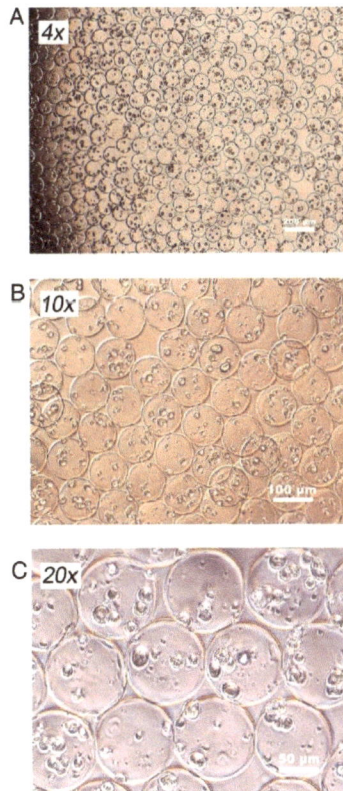

Figure 9: Morphology of C2C12-TGL-KDR cells encapsulated within 100 μm APA microcapsules. Optical microscopy at different magnifications. Scale bars are presented for each picture. Reproduced with permission from Ref. [45] © 2011 Elsevier.

5.1.2. Animals and Surgical Procedures

After anesthetization, a craniotomy is performed in each brain hemisphere [brain coordinates (from bregma): 0.6mm posterior and 1.1mm lateral]. In animals receiving microcapsule implants, the dura mater is excised, and 20 to 30 microcapsules are placed in the craniotomy, resulting in a bed of alginate microcapsules directly overlying the cerebral cortex. A small piece of surgical cellulose is placed over the microcapsules before suturing animals receiving microencapsulated cells (Fig. **10**).

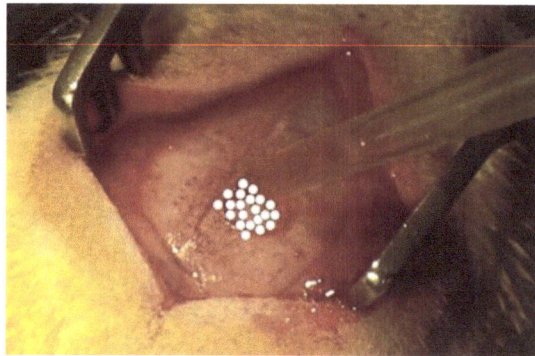

Figure 10: Craniotomy and microcapsule implantation in the brain. Reproduced with permission from © Biomaterials 2010; 31: 9373-9381, Elsevier.

ACKNOWLEDGEMENTS

This review is fully dedicated to Ainhoa Murua. We truly feel her loss and we will always keep her in our minds and hearts. T. López thanks the Basque Government (Department of Education, Universities and Research) for the fellowship grant.

CONFLICT OF INTEREST

The author(s) confirm that this chapter content has no conflict of interest.

REFERENCES

[1]   Orive G, Anitua E, Pedraz JL, Emerich DF. Biomaterials for promoting brain protection, repair and regeneration. Nat Rev Neurosci 2009; 10: 682-692.
[2]   Zhang J, Giesert F, Kloos K, Vogt Weisenhorn DM, Aigner L, Wurst W, Couillard-Despres S. A powerful transgenic tool for fate mapping and functional analysis of newly generated neurons. BMC Neurosci 2010; 11: 158-171.

[3]   Moris G, Vega JA. Factores neurotróficos: fundamentos para su aplicación clínica. Neurologia 2003; 18: 18-28.

[4]   Fumagalli F, Molteni R, Calabrese F, Maj PF, Racagni G, Riva MA. Neurotrophic factors in neurodegenerative disorders: potential for therapy. CNS Drugs 2008; 22: 1005-1019.

[5]   Portero A, Orive G, Hernández RM, Pedraz JL. Encapsulación de células para el tratamiento de enfermedades del sistema nervioso central. Rev Neurol 2010; 50 (7): 409-419.

[6]   Emerich DF, Orive G. Nanoparticle-Based Technologies for Treating and Imaging Brain Tumors. Current Cancer Drug Targets 2011; in press.

[7]   Pardridge WM. Molecular biology of the blood-brain barrier. Mol Biotechnol 2005; 30: 57-70.

[8]   Pardridge WM. The blood-brain barrier: bottleneck in brain drug development. NeuroRx 2005; 2: 3-14.

[9]   Pardridge WM. Brain drug targeting: the future of brain drug development. Cambridge, UK: Cambridge University Press; 2001.

[10]   Popovic N, Brundin P. Therapeutic potential of controlled drug delivery systems in neurodegenerative disorders. Int J Pharm 2006; 314: 120–126.

[11]   Denora N, Trapani A, Laquintana V, Lopedota A, Trapani G. Recent advances in medicinal chemistry and pharmaceutical technology strategies for drug delivery to the brain. Curr Topics Med Chem 2009; 9: 182–196.

[12]   Sahoo SK, Labhasetwar V. Nanotech approaches to drug delivery and imaging. Drug Discov Today 2003; 8: 1112–1120.

[13]   Schnyder A, Huwyler J. Drug transport to brain with targeted liposomes. NeuroRx 2005; 2: 99–107.

[14]   Lockman PR, Mumper RJ, Khan MA, Allen DD. Nanoparticle technology for drug delivery across the blood-brain barrier. Drug Dev Ind Pharm 2002; 28: 1–13.

[15]   Blasi P, Giovagnoli S, Schoubben A, Ricci M, Rossi C. Solid lipid nanoparticles for targeted brain drug delivery. Adv Drug Del Rev 2007; 59: 454–477.

[16]   Kaur IP, Bhandari R, Bhandari S, Kakkar V. Potential of solid lipid nanoparticles in brain drug targeting. J Control Release 2008; 127: 97–109.

[17]   Barinaga M. Neurotrophic factors enter the clinic. Science 1994; 264: 772–774.

[18]   Miller RG, Petajan JH, Bryan WW, Armon C, Barohn RJ, Goodpasture JC, Hoagland RJ, Parry GJ, Ross MA, Stromatt SC. A placebo-controlled trial of recombinant human ciliary neurotrophic (rhCNTF) factor in amyotrophic lateral sclerosis. rhCNTF ALS Study Group. Ann Neurol 1996; 39: 256–260.

[19]   Murua A, Portero A, Orive G, Hernández RM, De Castro M, Pedraz JL. Cell microencapsulation technology: Towards clinical application. J Control Release 2008; 132: 76-83.

[20]   Karp JM, Langer R. Development and therapeutic applications of advanced biomaterials. Curr Opin Biotechnol 2007; 18(5): 454-459.

[21]   Orive G, Hernández RM, Gascón AR, Pedraz JL. Challenges in cell encapsulation. Applications of Cell Immobilisation Biotechnology. Focus on Biotechnology In Nedović V, Willaert R, Eds. Applications of cell immobilisation biotechnology. Amsterdam, Springer, 2005; 8B, Part 2; pp. 185-196.

[22]   Lim F, Sun AM. Microencapsulated islets as bioartificial endocrine pancreas. Science 1980; 210: 908–910.

[23] Elliot RB, Escobar L, Calafiore R, Basta G, Garkavenko O, Vasconcellos A, Bambra C. Transplantation of micro- and macroencapsulated piglet islets into mice and monkeys. Transplant Proc 2005; 37: 466–469.

[24] Elliot RB, Escobar L, Tan PLJ, Garkavenko O, Calafiore R, Basta P, Vasconcellos AV, Emerich DF, Thanos C, Bambra C. Intraperitoneal alginate alginateencapsulated neonatal porcine islets in a placebo-controlled study with 16 diabetic cynomolgus primates. Transplant Proc 2005; 37: 3505–3508.

[25] Zilberman Y, Turgeman G, Pelled G, Xu N, Moutsatsos IK, Hortelano G, Gazit D. Polymer-encapsulated engineered adult mesenchymal stem cells secrete exogenously regulated rhBMP-2, and induce osteogenic and angiogenic tissue formation. Polym Adv Technol 2002; 13: 863–870.

[26] Paek HJ, Campaner AB, Kim JL, Golden L, Aaron RK, Ciombor DM, Morgan JR, Lysaght MJ. Microencapsulated cells genetically modified to overexpress human transforming growth factor-β1: viability and functionality in allogeneic and xenogeneic implant models. Tissue Eng 2006; 12: 1733–1739.

[27] Grellier M, Granja PL, Fricain J, Bidarra SJ, Renard M, Bareille R, Bourget C, Amédée J, Barbosa MA. The effect of the co-immobilization of human osteoprogenitors and endothelial cells within alginate microspheres on mineralization in a bone defect. Biomaterials 2009; 30: 3271–3278.

[28] Teng H, Zhang Y, Wang W, Ma X, Fei J. Inhibition of tumor growth in mice by endostatin derived from abdominal transplanted encapsulated cells. Acta Biochim Biophys Sin 2007; 39: 278–284.

[29] Löhr M, Müller P, Karle P, Stange J, Mitzner S, Jesnowski R, Nizze H, Nebe B, Liebe S, Salmons B, Gunzburg WH. Targeted chemotherapy by intratumour injection of encapsulated cells engineered to produce CYP2B1, an ifosfamide activating cytochrome P450. Gene Ther 1998; 5: 1070–1078.

[30] Goren A, Dahan N, Goren E, Baruch L, Machluf M. Encapsulated human mesenchymal stem cells: a unique hypoimmunogenic platform for long-term cellular therapy. FASEB J 2010; 24: 22–31.

[31] Madeddu P. Therapeutic angiogenesis and vasculogenesis for tissue regeneration, Exp Physiol 2005; 90: 315–326.

[32] Jacobs J. Combating cardiovascular disease with angiogenic therapy. Drug Discov Today 2007; 12: 1040–1045.

[33] Zang H, Zhu SJ, Wang W, Wey YJ, Hu SS. Transplantation of microencapsulated genetically modified xenogenic cells augments angiogenesis and improves heart function. Gene Ther 2008; 15: 40–48.

[34] Orive G, de Castro M, Ponce S, Hernández RM, Gascón AR, Bosch M, Alberch J, Pedraz JL. Long-term expression of erythropoietin from myoblasts immobilized in biocompatible and neovascularized microcapsules. Mol Ther 2005; 12: 283–289.

[35] Murua A, de Castro M, Orive G, Hernández RM, Pedraz JL. *In vitro* characterization and *in vivo* functionality of erythropoietin-secreting cells immobilized in alginate–poly-L-lysine–alginate microcapsules, Biomacromolecules 2007; 8: 3302–3307.

[36] Ponce S, Orive G, Hernández RM, Gascón AR, Canals JM, Muñoz MY, Pedraz JL. *In vivo* evaluation of EPO-secreting cells immobilized in different alginate–PLL microcapsules. J Control Release 2006; 116: 28–34.

[37]   Elliott RB, Escobar L, Tan PL, Muzina M, Zwine S, Buchanan C. Live encapsulated porcine islets from a type 1 diabetic patient 9.5 yr after xenotransplantation. Xenotransplantation 2007; 14: 157–161.

[38]   Löhr M, HoffmeyerA, Kröger J, Freund M, Hain J, Holle A, Karle P, Knofel WT, Liebe S, Muller P, Nizze H, Renner M, Saller RM, Wagner T, Hauenstein K, Günzburg WH, Salmons B. Microencapsulated cell-mediated treatment of inoperable pancreatic carcinoma. Lancet 2001; 357: 1591–1592.

[39]   Löhr JM, Kröger JC, Hoffmeyer A, Freund M, Hain J, Holle A, Knöfel WT, Liebe S, Nizze H, Renner M, Saller R, Müller P, Wagner T, Hauenstein K, Salmons B, Günzburg WH. Safety, feasibility and clinical benefit of localized chemotherapy using microencapsulated cells for inoperable pancreatic carcinoma in a phase I/II trial. Cancer Ther 2003; 1: 121–131.

[40]   Orive G, Gascón AR, Hernández RM, Igartua M, Pedraz JL. Cell microencapsulation technology for biomedical purposes: novel insights and challenges. Trends Pharmacol Sci 2003; 24: 207-210.

[41]   Orive G, Hernández RM, Gascón AR, Calafiore R, Chang TMS, De Vos P, Hortelano G, Hunkeler D, Lacík I, Pedraz JL. History, challenges and perspectives of cell microencapsulation. Trends Biotechnol 2004; 22: 87-92.

[42]   Aebischer P, Schluep M, Déglon N, Joseph JM, Hirt L, Heyd B, Goddard M, Hammang JP, Zurn AD, Kato AC, Regli F, Baetge EE. Intrathecal delivery of CNTF using encapsulated genetically modified xenogeneic cells in amyotrophic lateral sclerosis patients. Nat Med 1996; 2: 696-699.

[43]   Sajadi A, Bensadoun JC, Schneider BL, Lo Bianco C, Aebischer P. Transient Striatal delivery of GDNF *via* encapsulated cells leads to sustained behavioural improvement in a bilateral model of Parkinson disease. Neurobiol Dis 2006; 22; 119-129.

[44]   Zurn AD, Henry H, Schluep M, Aubert V, Winkel L, Eilers B, Bachmann C, Aebischer P. Evaluation of an intrathecal immune response in amyotrophic lateral sclerosis patients implanted with encapsulated genetically engineered xenogeneic cells. Cell Transplant 2000; 9: 471-484.

[45]   Santos E, Orive G, Calvo A, Catena R, Fernández-Robredo P, Layana AG, Hernández RM, Pedraz JL. Optimization of 100 μm alginate-poly-l-lysine-alginate capsules for intravitreous administration. J Control Release 2011; in press.

[46]   Murua A, Herran E, Orive G, Igartua M, Blanco FJ, Pedraz JL, Hernández RM. Design of a composite drug delivery system to prolong functionality of cell-based scaffolds. Int J Pharm 2011; 407(1-2): 142-150.

[47]   Catena R, Santos E, Orive G, Hernández RM, Pedraz JL, Calvo A. Improvement of the monitoring and biosafety of encapsulated cells using the SFGNESTGL triple reporter system. J Control Release 2010; 146(1): 93-98.

[48]   www.neurotechusa.com.

[49]   De Vos P, Bucko M, Gemeiner P, Navrátil M, Svitel J, Faas M, Strand BL, Skjak-Braek G, Morch YA, Vikartovská A, Lacík I, Kollárikavá G, Orive G, Poncelet D, Pedraz JL, Ansorge-Schumacher M B. Multiscale requirements for bioencapsulation in medicine and biotechnology. Biomaterials 2009; 30: 2559-2570.

[50]   Orive G, Hernández RM, Gascón AR, Calafiore R, Chang TMS, De Vos P, Hortelano G, Hunkeler D, Lacík I, Shapiro AM, Pedraz JL. Cell encapsulation: promise and progress. Nat Med 2003; 9: 104-107.

[51]   van der Laan LJ, Lockey C, Griffeth BC, Frasier FS, Wilson CA, Onions DE, Hering BJ, Long Z, Otto E, Torbett BE, *et al.* Infection by porcine endogenous retrovirus after islet xenotransplantation in SCID mice. Nature 2000; 407: 90–94.

[52]   Blusch JH, Patience C, Martin U. Pig endogenous retroviruses and xenotransplantation. Xenotransplantation 2002; 9 (4): 242-51.

[53]   Poncelet AJ, Denis D, Gianello P. Cellular xenotransplantation. Curr Opin Organ Transplant 2009; 14: 168-174.

[54]   Govan JRW, Fyfe JAM, Jarman TR. Isolation of alginate-producing mutants of Pseudomonas fluorescens, Pseudomonas putida and Pseudomonas mendocina. J Gen Microbiol 1981; 125: 217–220.

[55]   Hernandez RM, Orive G, Murua A, Pedraz JL. Microcapsules and microcarriers for *in situ* cell delivery; Advanced drug delivery reviews 2010; 62: 711-730.

[56]   Sakai S, Kawabata K, Ono T, Ijima H, Kawakami K. Development of mammalian cell-enclosing subsieve-size agarose capsules (< 100 μm) for cell therapy. Biomaterials 2005; 26: 4786–4792.

[57]   Santos E, Zarate J, Orive G, Hernández RM, Pedraz JL. Biomaterials in cell microencapsulation. In Pedraz JL, Orive G, Eds. Therapeutic applications of cell microencapsulation. Austin, Landes Bioscience, 2010; pp. 5-21.

[58]   Yamada KM. Adhesive recognition sequences. J Biol Chem 1991; 266: 12809–12812.

[59]   Ruoslahti E. RGD and other recognition sequences for integrins. Annu Rev Cell Dev Biol 1996; 12: 697–715.

[60]   Pinkse GG, Bouwman WP, Jiawan-Lalai R, Terpstra OT, Bruijn JA, de Heer E. Integrin signaling *via* RGD peptides and anti-beta1 antibodies confers resistance to apoptosis in islets of Langerhans, Diabetes 2006; 55: 312–317.

[61]   Rowley JA, Madlambayan G, Mooney DJ. Alginate hydrogels as synthetic extracellular matrix materials. Biomaterials 1999; 20: 45–53.

[62]   Augst AD, Kong HJ, Mooney DJ. Alginate hydrogels as biomaterials. Macromol Biosci 2006; 6: 623–633.

[63]   Di Giovanni G, Di Matteo V, Ennio E. Birth, Life and Death of Dopaminergic Neurons in the Substantia Nigra, Verlag/Wien, Springer 2009.

[64]   Linder MD, Plone MA, Mullins TD, Winn SR, Chandonait SE, Stott JA, Blaney TJ, Sherman SS, Emerich DF. Somatic delivery of catecholamines in the striatum attenuates Parkinosnian symptoms and widens the therapeutic window of oral Sinemet in rats. Exp Neurol 1997; 145: 130-140.

[65]   Lindner MD, Emerich DF. Therapeutic potential of a polymer-encapsulated L-DOPA and dopamine-producing cell line in rodent and primate models of Parkinson´s disease. Cell Transplant 1998; 7: 165-174.

[66]   Mínguez-Castellanos A, Escamilla-Sevilla F. Terapia celular y otras estrategias neurorregenerativas en la enfermedad de Parkinson (I). Rev Neurol 2005; 41: 604-614.

[67]   Lin LF, Doherty DH, Lile JD, Bektesh S, Collins F. GDNF: a glial cell line-derived neurotrophic factor for midbrain dopaminergic neurons. Science 1993; 260: 1130–1132.

[68]   Nutt JG, Burchiel KJ, Comella CL, Jankovic J, Lang AE, Laws Jr. ER, Lozano AM, Penn RD, Simpson Jr. RK, Stacy M,Wooten GF. Randomized, double-blind trial of glial cell line-derived neurotrophic factor (GDNF) in PD. Neurology 2003; 60: 69–73.

[69]   Kordower JH, Palfi S, Chen EY, Ma SY, Sendera T, Cochran EJ, Mufson EJ, Penn R, Goetz CG, Comella CD. Clinicopathological findings after intraventricular glial-derived

neurotrophic factor treatment in a patient with Parkinson's disease. Ann Neurol 1999; 46: 419–424.

[70]   Gill SS, Patel NK, Hotton GR, O'Sullivan K, McCarter R, Bunnage M, Brooks DJ, Svendsen CN, Heywood P. Direct brain infusion of glial cell line-derived neurotrophic factor in Parkinson disease. Nat Med 2003; 9: 589–595.

[71]   Slevin JT, Gerhardt GA, Smith CD, Gash DM, Kryscio R, Young B. Improvement of bilateral motor functions in patients with Parkinson disease through the unilateral intraputaminal infusion of glial cell linederived eurotrophic factor. J Neurosurg 2005; 102: 216–222.

[72]   Slevin JT, Gash DM, Smith CD, Gerhardt GA, Kryscio R, Chebrolu H, Walton A, Wagner R, Young AB. Unilateral intraputamenal glial cell line-derived neurotrophic factor in patients with Parkinson disease: response to 1 year of treatment and 1 year of withdrawal. J Neurosurg 2007; 106: 614–620.

[73]   Sajadi A, Bensadoun JC, Schneider BL, Lo Bianco C, Aebischer P. Transient striatal delivery of GDNF *via* encapsulated cells leads to sustained behavioural improvement in a bilateral model of Parkinson disease. Neurobiol Dis 2006; 22: 119-129.

[74]   Grandoso L, Ponce S, Manuel I, Arrúe A, Ruiz-Ortega JA, Ulibarri I, *et al.* Long-term survival of encapsulated GDNF secreting cells implanted within the striatum of parkinsonized rats. Int J Pharm 2007; 343: 69-78.

[75]   Date I, Shingo T, Yoshida H, Fujiwara K, Kobayashi K, Takeuchi A, Ohmoto T. Grafting of encapsulated genetically modified cells secreting GDNF into the striatum of parkinsonian model rats. Cell Transplant 2001; 10: 397-401.

[76]   Shingo T, Date I, Yoshida H, Ohmoto T. Neuroprotective and restorative effects of intrastriatal grafting of encapsulated GDNF-producing cells in a rat model of Parkinson's disease. J Neurosci Res 2002; 69: 946-54.

[77]   Yasuhara T, Shingo T, Muraoka K, Kobayashi K, Takeuchi A, Yano A, Wenji Y, Kameda M, Matsui T, Miyoshi Y, Date I. Early transplantation of an encapsulated glial cell line-derived neurotrophic factor-producing cell demonstrating strong neuroprotective effects in a rat model of Parkinson disease. J Neurosurg 2005; 102: 80-89.

[78]   Kishima H, Poyot T, Bloch J, Dauguet J, Condé F, Dollé F, Hinnen F, Pralong W, Palfi S, Déglon N, Aebischer P, Hantraye P. Encapsulated GDNF-producing C2C12 cells for Parkinson's disease: a pre-clinical study in chronic MPTP-treated baboons. Neurobiol Dis 2004; 16: 428-439.

[79]   Yasuhara T, Shingo T, Kobayashi K, Takeuchi A, Yano A, Muraoka K, Matsui T, Miyoshi Y, Hamada H, Date I. Neuroprotective effects of vascular endothelial growth factor (VEGF) upon dopaminergic neurons in a rat model of Parkinson's disease. Eur J Neurosci 2004; 19: 1494-504.

[80]   Yasuhara T, Shingo T, Muraoka K, Kameda M, Agari T, Wen Ji Y, Hayase H, Hamada H, Borlongan CV, Date I. Neurorescue effects of VEGF on a rat model of Parkinson's disease. Brain Res 2005; 1053: 10-18.

[81]   Yasuhara T, Shingo T, Muraoka K, Wen Ji Y, Kameda M, Takeuchi A, Yano A, Nishio S, Matsui T, Miyoshi Y, Hamada H, Date I. The differences between high and low dose administration of VEGF to dopaminergic neurons of *in vitro* and *in vivo* Parkinson's disease. Brain Res 2005; 1038: 1-10.

[82]   Date I, Shingo T, Yoshida H, Fujiwara K, Kobayashi K, Ohmoto T. Grafting of encapsulated dopamine-secreting cells in Parkinson's disease: long-term primate study. Cell Transplant 2000; 9: 705-709.

[83]   Zhang HL, Wu JJ, Ren HM, Wang J, Su YR, Jiang YP. Therapeutic effect of microencapsulated porcine retinal pigmented epithelial cells transplantation on rat model of Parkinson's disease. Neurosci Bull 2007; 23: 137-44.

[84]   Aebischer P, Tresco PA, Sagen J, Winn SR. Transplantation of microencapsulated bovine chromaffin cells reduces lesion-induced rotational asymmetry in rats. Brain Res 1991; 560: 43–49.

[85]   Date I, Shingo T, Ohmoto T, Emerich DF. Long-termenhanced chromaffin cell survival and behavioural recovery in hemiparkinsonian rats with co-grafted polymer-encapsulated human NGF-secreting cells. Exp Neurol 1997; 147: 10–17.

[86]   Mínguez-Castellanos A, Escamilla-Sevilla F. Terapia celular y otras estrategias neurorregenerativas en la enfermedad de Parkinson (II). Rev Neurol 2005; 41: 684-93.

[87]   Emgard M, Karlsson J, Hansson O, Brundin P. Patterns of cell death and dopaminergic neuron survival in intrastriatal nigral grafts. Exp Neurol 1999; 160: 279-88.

[88]   Sortwell CE, Pitzer MR, Collier TJ. Time course of apoptotic cell death within mesencephalic cell suspension grafts: implications for improving grafted dopamine neuron survival. Exp Neurol 2000; 165: 268-77.

[89]   Sautter J, Tseng JL, Braguglia D, Aebischer P, Spenger C, Seiler RW, Widmer HR, Zurn AD. Implants of polymer-encapsulated genetically modified cells releasing glial cell line-derived neurotrophic factor improve survival, growth, and function of fetal dopaminergic grafts. Exp Neurol 1998; 149: 230-236.

[90]   Ahn YH, Bensadoun JC, Aebischer P, Zurn AD, Seiger A, Björklund A, Lindvall O, Wahlberg L, Brundin P, Kaminski Schierle GS. Increased fiber outgrowth from xenotransplanted human embryonic dopaminergic neurons with co-implants of polymer-encapsulated genetically modified cells releasing glial cell line-derived neurotrophic factor. Brain Res Bull 2005; 66: 135-42.

[91]   Stover NP, Watts RL. Spheramine for treatment of Parkinson's disease. Neurotherapeutics 2008; 5: 252-259.

[92]   Falk T, Zhang S, Sherman SJ. Pigment epithelium derived factor (PEDF) is neuroprotective in two *in vitro* models of Parkinson's disease. Neurosci Lett 2009; 458: 49-52.

[93]   The Huntington's Disease Collaborative Research Group. A novel gene containing a trinucleotide repeat that is expanded and unstable on Huntington's disease chromosomes. Cell 1993; 72: 971–978.

[94]   Greenamyre JT, Shoulson I. Huntington's disease. In Calne D, Ed. Neurodegenerative Diseases. Saunders Press, Inc., Philadelphia, 1994; pp. 685–704.

[95]   Shoulson I. Huntington's disease: functional capacities in patients treated with neuroleptic and antidepressant drugs. Neurology 1981; 31: 1333–1335.

[96]   Emerich DF, Mooney DJ, Storrie H, Babu RS, Kordower JH. Injectable Hydrogels Providing Sustained Delivery of Vascular Endothelial Growth Factor are Neuroprotective in a Rat Model of Huntington's Disease. Neurotox Res 2010; 17: 66–74.

[97]   Emerich DF, Borlongan CV. Potential of Choroid Plexus Epithelial Cell Grafts for Neuroprotection in Huntington's Disease: What Remains Before Considering Clinical Trials. Neurotox Res 2009; 15: 205–211.

[98]   Emerich DF, Skinner SJM, Borlongan CV, Vasconcellos A, Thanos CG. The choroid plexus in the rise, fall, and repair of the brain, BioEssays 2005; 27: 262–274.

[99]   Emerich DF, Thanos CG. *In vitro* culture duration does not impact the ability of encapsulated choroid plexus transplants to prevent neurological deficits in excitotoxinlesioned rats. Cell Transplant 2006; 15: 595-602.

[100] Borlongan CV, Skinner SJM, Geaney M, Vasconcellos AV, Elliot RB, Emerich DF. Neuroprotection by encapsulated horoid plexus in a rodent model of Huntington's disease. Neuroreport 2004; 15: 2521-2525.

[101] Borlogan CV, Skinner SJM, Geaney M, Emerich DF. Transplants of encapsulated rat c horoid plexus exert neuroprotection in a rodent model of Huntingtons disease. Cell Transplant 2007; 16: 987-992.

[102] Emerich DF, Thanos CG, Goddard M, Skinner SJM, Geany MS, Bell WJ, Bintz B, Schneider P, Chu Y, Babu RS, Borlongan CV, Boekelheide K, Hall S, Bryant B, Kordower JH. Extensive neuroprotection by choroid plexus transplants in excitotoxin lesioned monkeys. Neurobiol Dis 2006; 23: 471–480.

[103] Emerich DF, Winn SR, Hantraye PM, Peschanski M, Chen ER, Chu Y, McDermott P, Baetge EE, Kordower JH. Protective effect of encapsulated cells producing neurotrophic factor CNTF in a monkey model of Huntington's disease. Nature 1997; 386: 395-399.

[104] Mittoux V, Joseph JM, Conde F, Palfi S, Dautry C, Poyot T, Bloch J, Deglon N, Ouary S, Nimchinsky EA, Brouillet E, Hof PR, Peschanski M, Aebischer P. Restoration of cognitive and motor functions by ciliary neurotrophic factor in a primate model of Huntington's disease. Hum Gene Ther 2000; 11: 1177-1187.

[105] Bloch J, Bachoud-Lévi AC, Déglon N, Lefaucheur JP, Winkel L, Palfi S, Nguyen JP, Bourdet C, Gaura V, Remy P, Brugières P, Boisse MF, Baudic S, Cesaro P, Hantraye P, Aebischer P, Peschanski M. Neuroprotective gene therapy for Huntington's disease, using polymer-encapsulated cells engineered to secrete human ciliary neurotrophic factor: results of a phase I study. Hum Gene Ther 2004; 15: 968–975.

[106] Kordower JH, Isacson O, Emerich DF. Cellular delivery of trophic factors for the treatment of Huntington's disease. Is neuroprotection possible? Exp Neurol 1999; 159: 4-20.

[107] Winn SR, Hammang JP, Emerich DF, Lee A, Palmiter RD, Baetge EE. Polymer-encapsulated cells genetically modified to secrete human nerve growth factor promote the survival of axotomized septal cholinergic neurons. Proc Natl Acad Sci USA1994; 91: 23–28.

[108] Fjord-Larsen L, Kusk P, Tornøe J, Juliusson B, Torp M, Bjarkam CR, Nielsen MS, Handberg A, Sørensen JC, Wahlberg LU. Long-term delivery of nerve growth factor by encapsulated cell biodelivery in the Göttingen minipig basal forebrain. Mol Ther 2010; 18(12): 2164-2172.

[109] Garcia P, Youssef I, Utvik JK, Florent-Bechard S, Barthelemy V, Malaplate-Armand C, Kriem B, Stenger C, Koziel V, Olivier JL, Escanye MC, Hanse M, Allouche A, Desbene C, Yen FT, Bjerkvig R, Oster T, Niclou SP, Pillot T. Ciliary neurotrophic factor cell-based delivery prevents synaptic impairment and improves memory in mouse models of Alzheimer's disease. J Neurosci 2010; 30: 7516–7527.

[110] Perry T, Greig NH. The glucagon-like peptides: a new genre in therapeutic targets for intervention in Alzheimer's disease. J Alzheimers Dis 2002; 4: 487–496.

[111] Perry T, Lahiri DK, Sambamurti K, Chen D, Mattson MP, Egan JM, Greig NH. Glucagon-like peptide-1 decreases endogenous amyloid-beta peptide (Abeta) levels and protects hippocampal neurons from death induced by Abeta and iron. J Neurosci Res 2003; 72: 603–612.

[112] Perry T, Haughey NJ, Mattson MP, Egan JM, Greig NH. Protection and reversal of excitotoxic neuronal damage by glucagon-like peptide-1 and exendin-4. J Pharmacol Exp Ther 2002; 302: 881–888.

[113]   Klinge PM, Harmening K, Miller MC, Heile A, Wallrapp C, Geigle P, Brinker T. Encapsulated native and glucagon-like peptide-1 transfected human mesenchymal stem cells in a transgenic mouse model of Alzheimer's disease. Neuroscience Letters 2011; 497: 6–10.

[114]   Spuch C, Antequera D, Portero A, Orive G, Hernández RM, Molina JA, Bermejo-Pareja F, Pedraz JL, Carro E. The effect of encapsulated VEGF-secreting cells on brain amyloid load and behavioural impairment in a mouse model of Alzheimer's disease. Biomaterials 2010; 31: 5608-5618.

[115]   Antequera D, Portero A, Bolosa M, Orive G, Hernández RM, Pedraz JL, Carro E. Encapsulated VEGF-Secreting Cells Enhance Proliferation of Neuronal Progenitors in the Hippocampus of APP/Ps1 Mice. JAD 2012; 30: 1-14.

[116]   Emerich DF, Vasconcellos A. Cellular transplants, 20 years later: the pharma iniciative. Regen Med 2009; 4 (4): 485-487.

[117]   Lindvall O, Wahlberg LU. Encapsulated cell delivery of GDNF: a novel clinical strategy for neuroprotection and neurodegeneration in Parkinson's disease? Exp Neurol 2008; 209: 82-88.

[118]   www.nsgene.dk.

[119]   Rowland LP, Shneider NA. Amyotrophic lateral sclerosis. N Engl J Med 2001; 344 (22): 1688-1700.

[120]   Tan SA, Déglon N, Zurn AD, Baetge EE, Bamber B, Kato AC, Aebischer P. Rescue of motoneurons from axotomy-induced cell death by polymer encapsulated cells genetically engineered to release CNTF. Cell Transpl 1996; 5: 577–587.

[121]   Sagot Y, Tan SA, Baetge E, Schmalbruch H, Kato AC, Aebischer P. Polymer encapsulated cell lines genetically engineered to release ciliary neurotrophic factor can slow down progressive motor neuronopathy in the mouse. Eur J Neurosci 1995; 7: 1313–1322.

[122]   Deglon N, Heyd B, Tan SA, Joseph JM, Zurn AD, Aebischer P. Central nervous system delivery of recombinant ciliary neurotrophic factor by polymer encapsulated differentiated C2C12 myoblasts. Hum. Gene Ther 1996; 7: 2135–2146.

[123]   Zurn AD, Henry H, Schluep M, Aubert V, Winkel L, Eilers B, Bachmann C, Aebischer P. Evaluation of an intrathecal immune response in amyotrophic lateral sclerosis patients implanted with encapsulated genetically engineered xenogeneic cells. Cell Transplant 2000; 9: 471-484.

[124]   Aebischer P, Schluep M, Déglon N, Joseph JM, Hirt L, Heyd B, Goddard M, Hammang JP, Zurn AD, Kato AC, Regli F, Baetge EE. Intrathecal delivery of CNTF using encapsulated genetically modified xenogeneic cells in amyotrophic lateral sclerosis patients. Nat Med 1996; 2: 696-699.

[125]   Zheng C, Nennesmo I, Fadeel B, Henter JI. Vascular endothelial growth factor prolongs survival in a transgenic mouse model of ALS. Ann Neurol 2004; 56: 564–567.

[126]   Storkebaum E, Lambrechts D, Dewerchin M, Moreno-Murciano MP, Appelmans S, Oh H, Van Damme P, Rutten B, Man WY, De Mol M, Wyns S, Manka D, Vermeulen K, Van Den Bosch L, Mertens N, Schmitz C, Robberecht W, Conway EM, Collen D, Moons L, Carmeliet P. Treatment of motoneuron degeneration by intracerebroventricular delivery of VEGF in a rat model of ALS. Nat Neurosci 2005; 8: 85–92.

[127]   Mohajeri MH, Figlewicz DA, Bohn MC. Intramuscular grafts of myoblasts genetically modified to secrete glial cell line-derived neurotrophic factor prevent motoneuron loss and

disease progression in a mouse model of familial amyotrophic lateral sclerosis. Hum Gene Ther 1999; 10: 1853–1866.

[128] Suzuki M, McHugh J, Tork C, Shelley B, Hayes A, Bellantuono I, Aebischer P, Svendsen CN. Direct muscle delivery of GDNF with human mesenchymal stem cells improves motor neuron survival and function in a rat model of familial ALS. Mol Ther 2008; 16: 2002–2010.

[129] Katsuragi S, Ikeda T, Date I, Shingo T, Yasuhara T, Ikenoue T. Grafting of glial cell line-derived neurotrophic factor secreting cells for hypoxic-ischemic encephalopathy in neonatal rats. Am J Obstet Gynecol 2005; 192: 1137-1145.

[130] Katsuragi S, Ikeda T, Date I, Shingo T, Yasuhara T, Mishima K, Aoo N, Harada K, Egashira N, Iwasaki K, Fujiwara M, Ikenoue T. Implantation of encapsulated glial cell line-derived neurotrophic factor-secreting cells prevents long-lasting learning impairment following neonatal hypoxic-ischemic brain insult in rats. Am J Obstet Gynecol 2005; 192: 1028-1037.

[131] Borlongan CV, Skinner SJM, Geaney M, Vasconcellos AV, Elliot RB, Emerich DF. CNS grafts of rat choroid plexus protect against cerebral ischemia in adult rats. Neuroreport 2004; 15: 1543-1547.

[132] Borlongan CV, Skinner SJM, Geaney M, Vasconcellos AV, Elliot RB, Emerich DF. Intracerebral transplantation of porcine choroid plexus provides structural and functional neuroprotection in a rodent model of stroke. Stroke 2004; 35: 2206-2210.

[133] Yano A, Shingo T, Takeuchi A, Yasuhara T, Kobayashi K, Takahashi K, *et al.* Encapsulated vascular endothelial growth factor-secreting cell grafts have neuroprotective and angiogenic effects on focal cerebral ischemia. J Neurosurg 2005; 103: 104-114.

[134] Heile A, Brinker T. Clinical translation of stem cell therapy in traumatic brain injury: the potential of encapsulated mesenchymal cell biodelivery of glucagon-like peptide-1. Dialogues Clin Neurosci 2011; 13(3): 279-286.

[135] Kim D, Schallert T, Liu Y, Browarak T, Nayeri N, Tessler A, Fischer I, Murray M. Transplantation of genetically modified fibroblasts expressing BDNF in adult rats with subtotal hemisection improves specific motor and sensory functions. Neurorehabil Neural Repair 2001; 15: 141–150.

[136] Liu Y, Kim D, Himes BT, Chow SY, Schallert T, Murray M, Tessler A, Fischer I. Transplants of fibroblasts genetically modified to Express BDNF promote regeneration of adult rat rubrospinal axons and recovery of forelimb function. J Neurosci 1999; 19: 4370–4387.

[137] Tobias CA, Han SSW, Shumsky JS, Kim D, Tumolo M, Dhoot NO, Wheatley MA, Fisher I, Tessler A, Murray M. Alginate encapsulated BDNF-producing fibroblast grafts permit recovery of function alter spinal cord injury in the absence of immune suppression. J Neurotrauma 2005; 22: 138–156.

[138] http://clinicaltrials.gov/ct2/show/NCT01298830

[139] Czech KA, Sagen J. Update on cellular transplantation into the rat CNS as a novel therapy for chronic pain. Prog Neurobiol 1995; 46: 507–515.

[140] Sagen J, Pappas GD, Pollard HB. Analgesia induced by isolated bovine chromaffin cells implanted in rat spinal cord. Proc Natl Acad Sci USA 1986; 83: 7522–7526.

[141] Sagen J, Wang H, Tresco PA, Aebischer P: Transplants of immunologically isolated xenogeneic chromaffin cells provide a long-term source of pain reducing neuroactive substances. J Neurosci 1993; 13: 2415-2423.

[142] Buchser E, Goddard M, Heyd B, Joseph JM, Favre J, de Tribolet N, Lysaght M, Aebischer P. Immunoisolated xenogenic chromaffin cell therapy for chronic pain. Initial clinical experience. Anesthesiology 1996; 85: 1005-1012.

[143] Jeon Y, Kwak K, Kim S, Kim Y, Lim J, Baek W. Intrathecal implants of microencapsulated xenogenic chromaffin cells provide a long-term source of analgesic substances. Transplant Proc 2006; 38: 3061–3065.

[144] Jeon Y, Baek WY, Chung SH, Shin N, Kim HR, Lee SA. Cultured human chromaffin cells grafted in spinal subarachnoid space relieves allodynia in a pain rat model. Korean J Anesthesiol 2011; 60(5): 357-361.

[145] Wu S, Ma C, Li G, Mai M, Wu Y. Intrathecal implantation of microencapsulated PC12 cells reduces cold allodynia in a rat model of neuropathic pain. Artif Organs 2011; 35(3): 294-300.

[146] Read TA, Stensvaag V, Vindenes H, Ulvestad E, Bjerkvig R, Thorsen F. Cells encapsulated in alginate:a potential system for delivery of recombinant proteins to malignant brain tumours. Int J Dev Neurosci 1999; 17: 653-663.

[147] Visted T, Lund-Johansen M. Progress and challenges for cell encapsulation in brain tumour therapy. Exp Opin Biol Ther 2003; 3: 551-561.

[148] Visted T, Bjerkvig R, Enger PO. Cell encapsulation technology as a therapeutic strategy for CNS malignancies. Neuro Oncol 2001; 3(3): 201-210.

[149] Cirone P, Bourgeois JM, Austin RC, Chang PL. A novel approach to tumor suppression with microencapsulated recombinant cells. Hum Gene Ther 2002; 13: 1157–1166.

[150] Sabel MS, Arora A, Su G, Mathiowitz E, Reineke JJ, Chang AE. Synergistic effect of intratumoral IL-12 and TNF-α microspheres: systemic anti-tumor immunity is mediated by both CD8+ CTL and NK cells. Surgery 2007; 142: 749–760.

[151] Hao S, Su L, Guo X *et al.* A novel approach to tumor suppression using microencapsulated engineered J558/TNF-alpha cells. Exp Oncol 2005; 27:56-60.

[152] Moran DM, Koniaris LG, Jablonski EM *et al.* Microencapsulation of engineered cells to deliver sustained high circulating levels of interleukin-6 to study hepatocellular carcinoma progression. Cell Transplant 2006; 15:785-798.

[153] Pelegrin M, Marin M, Noel D *et al.* Systemic long-term delivery of antibodies in immunocompetent animals using cellulose sulphate capsules containing antibody-producing cells. Gene Ther 1998; 5:828-834.

[154] Dautzenberg H, Schuldt U, Grasnick G *et al.* Development of cellulose sulfate-based polyelectrolyte complex microcapsules for medical applications. Ann N Y Acad Sci 1999; 875:46-63.

[155] Pelegrin M, Marin M, Oates A *et al.* Immunotherapy of a viral disease by *in vivo* production of therapeutic monoclonal antibodies. Hum Gene Ther 2000; 11:1407-1415.

[156] Dubrot J, Portero A, Orive G, Hernández RM, Palazón A, Rouzaut A, Perez-Gracia JL, Hervás-Stubbs S, Pedraz JL, Melero I. Delivery of immunostimulatory monoclonal antibodies by encapsulated hybridoma cells. Cancer immunol immunother. 2010; 59 (11): 1621-31.

[157] Kuijlen JM, de Haan BJ, Helfrich W, de Boer JF, Samplonius D, Mooij JJ, de Vos P. The efficacy of alginate encapsulated CHO-K1 single chain-TRAIL producer cells in the treatment of brain tumors. J Neurooncol 2006; 78(1): 31-39.

[158] Read T, Sorensen DR, Mahesparan R, Enger PØ, Timpl R, Olsen BR, Hjelstuen MHB, Haraldseth O, Bjerkvig R. Local endostatin treatment of gliomas administered by microencapsulated producer cells, Nat Biotechnol 2001; 19 29–34.

[159] Joki T, Machluf M, Atala A, Zhu J, Seyfried NT, Dunn IF, Abe T, Carroll RS, Black PM. Continuous release of endostatin from microencapsulated engineered cells for tumor therapy. Nat Biotechnol 2001; 19: 35–39.

[160] Bjerkvig R, Read TA, Vajkoczy P, Aebischer P, Pralong W, Platt S, Melvik JE, Hagen A, Dornish M. Cell therapy using encapsulated cells producing endostatin. Acta Neurochir Suppl 2003; 88: 137-141.

[161] Goren A, Dahan N, Goren E, Baruch L, Machluf M. Encapsulated human mesenchymal stem cells: a unique hypoimmunogenic platform for long-term cellular therapy. FASEB J 2010; 24: 22–31.

[162] Cirone P, Bourgeois JM, Chang PL. Antiangiogenic cancer therapy with microencapsulated cells. Hum Gene Ther 2003; 14: 1065-1077.

[163] Li AA, Shen F, Zhang T *et al.* Enhancement of myoblast microencapsulation for gene therapy. J Biomed Mater Res B Appl Biomater 2006; 77: 296-306.

[164] Cirone P, Bourgeois JM, Shen F, Chang PL. Combined immunotherapy and antiangiogenic therapy of cancer with microencapsulated cells. Hum Gene Ther 2004; 15: 945–959.

[165] Cirone P, Shen F, Chang PL. A multiprong approach to cancer gene therapy by coencapsulated cells. Cancer Gene Ther 2005; 12: 369–380.

[166] Salmons B, Gunzburg WH. Therapeutic application of cell microencapsulation in cancer. In Orive G, Pedraz JL, Eds. Therapeutic applications of cell microencapsulation. Austin, Landes Bioscience, 2010; pp. 92–103.

[167] Löhr M, Hoffmeyer A, Kröger J, Freund M, Hain J, Holle A, Karle P, Knofel WT, Liebe S, Muller P, Nizze H, Renner M, Saller RM, Wagner T, Hauenstein K, Gunzburg WH, Salmons B. Microencapsulated cell-mediated treatment of inoperable pancreatic carcinoma. Lancet 2001; 357: 1591–1592.

[168] Löhr JM, Kröger JC, Hoffmeyer A, Freund M, Hain J, Holle A, Knöfel WT, Liebe S, Nizze H, Renner M, Saller R, Müller P, Wagner T, Hauenstein K, Salmons B, Günzburg WH. Safety, feasibility and clinical benefit of localized chemotherapy using microencapsulated cells for inoperable pancreatic carcinoma in a phase I/II trial. Cancer Ther 2003; 1: 121–131.

[169] Salmons B, Hauser O, Günzburg WH, Tabotta W. GMP production of an encapsulated cell therapy product: Issues and considerations. BioProcessing Journal 2007; 6 (2): 37-44.

[170] Levi-Montalcini R, Ed. Neurological Disorders: Public Health Challenges, WHO Press. Geneva, 2007.

[171] Privitera M. Current challenges in the management of epilepsy. Am J Manag 2001; 910 (Care 17): S195–S203.

[172] Boison D. Adenosine augmentation therapies (AATs) for epilepsy: Prospect of cell and gene therapies. Epilepsy Research 2009; 85: 131-141.

[173] Boison D. Adenosine and epilepsy: from therapeutic rationale to new therapeutic strategies. Neuroscientist 2005; 11: 25-36.

[174] Lado FA, Moshe SL. How do seizures stop? Epilepsia 2008; 49: 1651-1664.

[175] Huber A, Padrun V, Deglon N, Aebischer P, Mohler H, Boison D. Grafts of adenosine-releasing cells suppress seizures in kindling epilepsy. Proc Natl Acad Sci USA. 2001; 98: 7611-7616.

[176] Güttinger M, Fedele DE, Koch P, Padrun V, Pralong W, Brüstle O, Boison D. Suppression of kindled seizures by paracrine adenosine release from stem cell derived brain implants. Epilepsia 2005a; 46,:1-8.

[177] Kanter-Schlifke I, Fjord-Larsen L, Kusk P, Ängehagen M, Wahlberg L, Kokaia M. GDNF released from encapsulated cells suppresses seizure activity in the epileptic hippocampus. Exp Neurol 2009; 216 (2): 413-419.

[178] Kuramoto S, Yasuhara T, Agari T, Kondo A, Jing M, Kikuchi Y, Shinko A, Wakamori T, Kameda M, Wang F, Kin K, Edahiro S, Miyoshi Y, Date I. BDNF-secreting capsule exerts neuroprotective effects on epilepsy model of rats. Brain Res 2011; 12; 1368: 281-289.

Send Orders of Reprints at reprints@benthamscience.net
Bioencapsulation of Living Cells for Diverse Medical Applications, 2013, 153-177   **153**

CHAPTER 6

Production of Cell-Enclosing Microparticles and Microcapsules Using a Water-Immiscible Fluid Under Laminar Flow and Its Applications in Cell Therapy

Shinji Sakai[1,*], Shinji Tanaka[2], Koei Kawakami[3] and Shigeki Arii[2]

[1]Division of Chemical Engineering, Department of Materials Science and Engineering, Graduate School of Engineering Science, Osaka University, Osaka, Japan; [2]Department of Chemical Engineering, Faculty of Engineering, Kyushu University, Fukuoka, Japan and [3]Department of Hepato-Biliary-Pancreatic Surgery, Tokyo Medical and Dental University, Graduate School of Medicine, Tokyo, Japan

Abstract: Reduction in the diameter of cell-enclosing spherical vehicles for cell therapy is an important issue, giving benefits such as higher molecular exchangeability between the enclosed cells and the ambient environment, higher mechanical stability and biocompatibility. In this chapter we review our recent studies for the production of cell-enclosing microparticles and microcapsules of about 100-200 μm in diameter. They are much smaller than conventional cell-enclosing spherical vehicles, which are typically between 300 and 1,000 μm in diameter. We prepare these small vehicles using droplet breakup through jetting in a water-immiscible liquid stream under laminar flow. Factors for controlling the size of droplets and methods for obtaining gelled vehicles are also described. In addition, we demonstrate the feasibility of these small vehicles for cell therapy by showing the results obtained after implanting the vehicles enclosing cells expressing a cancer-prodrug-converting-enzyme into a mouse with a subcutaneously formed tumor.

Keywords: Microcapsule, cell therapy, co-flowing stream, duplex microcapsule, alginate, agarose, gelatin, horseradish peroxidase, alginate lyase, cross-linking, enzyme, degradation, hollow core, hydrogel membrane, droplets breakup, water-immiscible fluid, alginate with phenolic moieties, hydrogen peroxide, laminar flow, subsieve-size capsule.

*Address correspondence to Shinji Sakai: Department of Materials Science and Engineering, Graduate School of Engineering Science, Osaka University, 1-3 Machikaneyama-cho, Toyonaka, Osaka 560-8531, Japan; Tel: +81-6-6850-6252; E-mail : sakai@cheng.es.osaka-u.ac.jp

1. INTRODUCTION

After the first successful report by Lim and Sun in 1980 [1], a wide variety of spherical vehicles has been developed for cell encapsulation. In particular, a large number of studies have been reported regarding enhancement of molecular permeability, mechanical stability and biocompatibility since these are crucial factors governing the successful therapeutic treatment after implantation [2-5]. These studies can be classified into two categories depending on the research approach. One category includes the advancement of vehicle-forming biomaterials [6-12] and the other includes adjustment and optimization of vehicle size [13-18]. Focusing on the size, the majority of reported cell-enclosing spherical vehicles have had diameters of several hundred micrometers to millimeters. This is because cell-encapsulation technology has been developed based on the technique originally developed for enclosing pancreatic insulin secretion tissues of 50-300 μm in diameter for the treatment of diabetes [1]. Recent advances in genetic engineering have enabled the use of single cells as reactors to produce desired proteins [19-21]. However, the vehicles originally developed for pancreatic tissues encapsulation have been used even for the encapsulation of single cells of less than 30 μm in diameter [22-24]. Taking into account the size of single cells, it can be recognized that conventional spherical vehicles are too large, *i.e.*, vehicles with a size suitable for single cell encapsulation should be used.

Reduction in vehicle size may make recovery from body more complex in the unlikely case where the capsules were to cause adverse effects, but beyond this, it may enable further practical applications in clinical studies. One positive effect is the enhancement of molecular exchangeability of species such as oxygen, nutrients and waste metabolites between enclosed cells and the surrounding environment [25, 26]. This also enables the rapid release of therapeutic substances. Rapid release into body fluids is attractive for therapeutic molecules with a short half-life. In addition, reduction in vehicle size should allow the use of immune-privileged sites for implantation, such as spleen capsules, the omental pouch or the liver through the portal vein. The most frequently used implantation site is the peritoneal cavity, because of the large available space. However, this is not the most efficient site in terms of immune molecule diffusion and vascularization [13]. Furthermore, smaller vehicles would reduce the size of the capsule injection device, thereby reducing surgical trauma and increase the alternative sites available for implantation [27]. It has also been reported that smaller spherical vehicles induced less foreign body response to the implanted vehicles [16]. In some studies, successful preparation of microcapsules of 100-200 μm has been reported [28-31] but development of smaller spherical vehicles for cell-encapsulation is a challenging issue even at present. In the industrial field, we can find a variety of methods for obtaining spherical vehicles around 100 μm in diameter. However, the majority of these are not applicable to mammalian cell encapsulation because of the sensitivity of the cells to temperature, pH, solvents and forces exerted by the external environment such as shear stress. In this chapter, we describe our approach to developing spherical vehicles that are smaller than conventional ones of more than 300 μm in diameter, using a droplet breakup technique in a water-immiscible liquid stream under laminar flow. In addition, we describe the potency of the vehicles for cell therapies based on our recent studies. In the following sections we refer to spherical vehicles with a solid core as "microparticles" and vehicles with a liquid core as "microcapsules".

2. DROPLET PRODUCTION IN WATER-IMMISCIBLE LAMINAR FLOW

The principle of our method for obtaining cell-enclosing droplets resulting in cell-enclosing microparticles after subsequent gelation is based on the breakup into droplets of an aqueous solution injected into an immiscible fluid stream flowing in the same direction (laminar flow). This system has been used for the preparation of cell-enclosing microparticles and microcapsules since the first report describing successful implantation of encapsulated tissues for treatment of diseases in 1980 [1]. In that report, pancreatic islets-enclosing calcium-alginate microparticles of 300-800 μm in diameter were prepared from islets suspended in a sodium-alginate aqueous solution by injecting the solution into an air flow, based on a method reported in 1969 [32], and subsequently collected in a solution containing calcium ions for gelation. Since the first report, the oldest but the most widely applied ambient fluid has been air [33-38]. The size of the cell-containing droplets can be controlled by changing the flow rate of the ambient air [39] as well as the size of the needle from which the cell-suspending aqueous solution is extruded and the flow rate of the aqueous solution. A limitation of the system is that it is impossible to obtain droplets with narrow size distribution that are smaller than the diameter of the needle from which the cell-suspending aqueous polymer solution is extruded [28, 39]. It may be thought that increasing the air flow rate decreases the size of the resultant droplets. This is partly true but the resultant droplets show a heterogeneous size distribution, the reason for which is the occurrence of fluctuations in air flow under the flow rate necessary for obtaining droplets that are smaller than the needle [40]. Even when using air as ambient fluid, cell-enclosing microparticles of around 100 μm in diameter and a narrow size distribution can be produced using a nozzle of several dozen micrometers in diameter from which cell-suspending solution is extruded [29, 41]. Such small nozzles can be prepared using microfabrication techniques. However, attention must be paid to the risk of the nozzle clogging or plugging with increasing viscosity of the extruded solution [42] and decreasing diameter of the nozzles. Without complete dispersion, the cells suspended in the aqueous solution themselves pose a risk of clogging and plugging the nozzle.

In our system, we use liquid paraffin as the water-immiscible ambient fluid. In addition, the liquid paraffin flows in tubules less than 2 mm in diameter. The droplet preparation device is composed of a syringe filled with a polymer aqueous solution containing cells and equipped with an inner needle (Fig. **1A**), an outer tubule **(B)**, and a reservoir of liquid paraffin from which liquid paraffin flows under gas pressure **(C)**. The inner needle is positioned upstream in the vicinity of a coaxial outer tubule through which the liquid paraffin flows. The resultant emulsion system or gelated particles are collected at the tip of the outer tubule **(D)**. From a hydrodynamics point of view, laminar flow is easily developed from the fluid with higher viscosity in a thinner tubule under the same flow rate. It would be easy to imagine that the constant force necessary for obtaining droplets with a narrow size distribution can be imposed on the cell-suspending solution for breakup into droplets in the co-flowing laminar flow. We first attempted to develop cell-enclosing microparticles with diameter less than 100 μm and a narrow size distribution using medical syringe needles with a diameter of several hundred micrometers to inject the cell-suspending solution. It should be noted at this point that the resultant system obtained from the droplets breakup technique is an emulsion system. For obtaining emulsion systems, magnetic stirrers and homogenizers are frequently used [43, 44]. These techniques are effective for preparing droplets of less than 100 μm in diameter but the droplets are heterogeneous in size. As shown in Fig. **2**, the droplets obtained by breakup in a liquid paraffin stream flowing under laminar flow show a narrow size distribution [45]. The size of the droplets is controllable by changing the flow rates of liquid paraffin and aqueous polymer solution (Fig. **3**) [45, 46] and the diameter of the needle (Fig. **4**) [46]. The viscosity of the polymer solution is also a factor governing the size of resultant droplets (Fig. **5**) [47]. A notable finding was that smaller droplets were obtained from a higher viscosity solution at a fixed flow rate of liquid paraffin [47]. This means vehicles with a higher mechanical strength can be obtained from a synergy of reduction in diameter and a tightening of microscopic structure of the gel, using a smaller quantity of ambient liquid paraffin. The smaller droplet generation from a higher viscosity solution is because of droplet breakup from a thinner ligament resulting from the higher viscosity (Fig. **6**). An important finding for mammalian cell-encapsulation applications is that cells enclosed in droplets less than 100 μm in diameter have virtually unhindered viability [46]. Furthermore, the cells retrieved from the droplets showed almost the same growth profiles in a cell culture dish as those seeded using a normal subculture protocol [47], despite the fact that mammalian cells are easily damaged by forces exerted by the external environment such as shear stress. Drag force has the most influence in cell damage. These findings demonstrate that the drag force necessary for obtaining droplets less than 100 μm in diameter is insufficient to damage cell viability and growth activity. We attribute the negligible harmful effect on living cells to the harmless droplet generation mode. Droplet generation in an immiscible liquid is classified into two different mechanisms: either the droplets are formed close to the capillary tip (dripping) or they break-off from an extended liquid ligament (jetting) [48]. The droplet break-off in our process giving droplets of around 100 μm in diameter is based on jetting. In this process, a coaxial ligament of cell-suspending aqueous polymer solution breaks off into segments that acquire a spherical shape. This phenomenon is explained by Rayleigh-Plateau hydrodynamic instability [49], in which interfacial tension between the aqueous solution and the liquid paraffin is the crucial force for the formation of droplets.

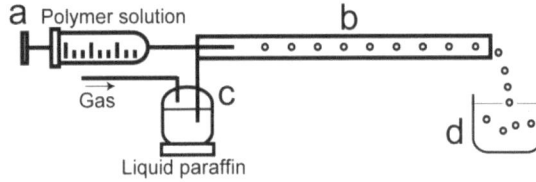

Figure 1: Schematic of the droplet production device composed of (A) a syringe equipped with a needle, (B) a tubule, (C) a liquid paraffin reservoir for flowing liquid paraffin under gas pressure, and (D) collector.

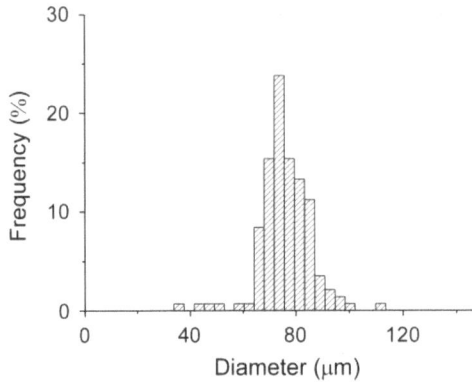

Figure 2: Frequency of agarose microparticle diameters under a condition whereby 4 wt% agarose solution was extruded at a velocity of 1.2 cm/sec into an immiscible coflowing liquid paraffin stream with a velocity of 20.8 cm/sec from a needle of 300 μm inner diameter. (Reproduced with permission from Sakai *et al.* Biomaterials [45] @2005 Elsevier).

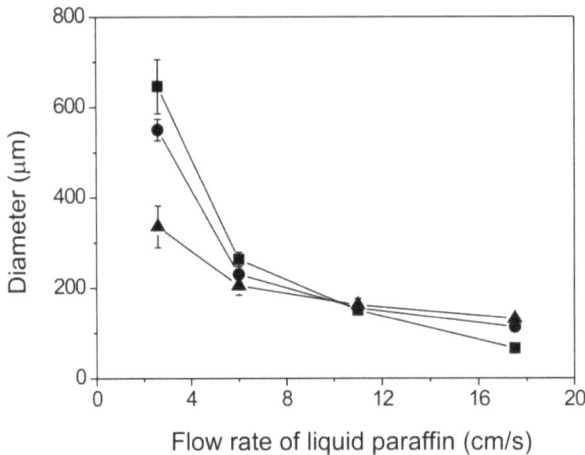

Figure 3: Droplet diameter as a function of liquid paraffin velocity for three different 2 wt% sodium alginate solution velocities: (■) 1.2 cm/s, (●) 2.6 cm/s, and (▲) 4.7 cm/s. A needle with 300 μm i.d., 480 μm o.d. was used. Bars: SDs. (Reproduced with permission from Sakai *et al.* Biotechnol Bioeng [46] @2004 Wiley Periodicals, Inc.).

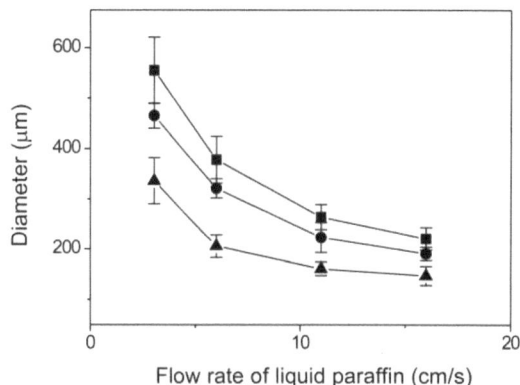

Figure 4: Droplet diameter as a function of the liquid paraffin flow rate for three needles of different diameters: (■) 940 μm i.d., 1200 μm o.d.; (●) 480 μm i.d., 700 μm o.d.; and (▲) 300 μm i.d., 480 μm o.d. Bars: SDs. (Reproduced with permission from Sakai *et al.* Biotechnol Bioeng [46]@2004 Wiley Periodicals, Inc.).

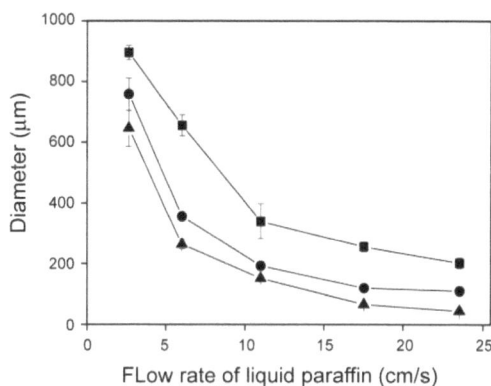

Figure 5: Droplet diameter as a function of the liquid paraffin velocity for three aqueous solutions differing in viscosity: (■) 1.0, (●) 36, and (▲) 194 mPa·s. Aqueous solutions were extruded at a velocity of 1.2 cm/s from a needle of 300 μm inner diameter. Bars: SDs. (Reproduced with permission from Sakai *et al.* Biotechnol Prog [47]@2005 American Institute of Chemical Engineers).

3. CELL ENCAPSULATION

A limitation of the droplet breakup technique using a water-immiscible liquid stream is that gelation of droplets has to be carried out in the water-immiscible liquid to obtain spherical vehicles. We prepared microparticles based on two types of gelation processes, thermal gelation using unmodified agarose [45, 50] and agarose-based materials [51, 52], and enzymatic gelation using alginate and cellulose incorporating phenolic hydroxyl groups [53, 54]. Since the 1980s, a variety of materials have been used for cell-enclosing microparticles and microcapsules [2, 3].

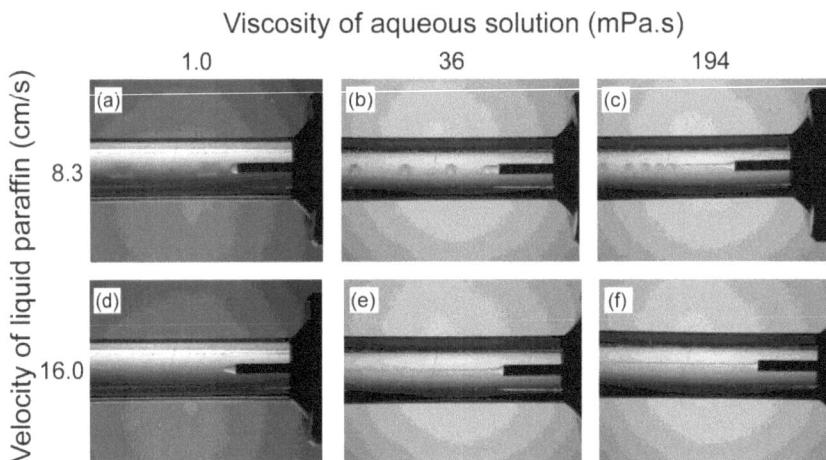

Figure 6: Three aqueous solutions of different viscosity, (a, d) 1 mPa·s, (b, e) 36 mPa·s, and (c, f) 194 mPa·s were extruded from a needle of 300 μm inner diameter into an ambient liquid paraffin stream at a velocity of 3.6 cm/s. The liquid paraffin flows from right to left at velocities of (a, b, c) 8.3 cm/s, and (d, e, f) 16.0 cm/s. (Reproduced with permission from Sakai *et al.* Biotechnol Prog [47]@2005 American Institute of Chemical Engineers).

3.1. Agarose Microparticles

Agarose is a natural thermosensitive polysaccharide extracted from the cell wall of agarophyte seaweed. Agarose with a gelling temperature between 15 and 30°C has been used for cell-immobilization in gels such as 3-D modeling [55] and tissue engineering [56-60] and for cell encapsulation in microparticles [61-63] because of the moderate sol-to-gel transition temperature for mammalian cells and high biocompatibility.

Agarose gel is obtained from an aqueous agarose solution prepared first by heating an aqueous suspension of agarose powder until a clear solution is formed. The solution is then cooled to around 37°C to allow suspension of living mammalian cells without hindrance from gelation of the solution. We filled a syringe equipped with a water jacket maintained at 37°C with suspension. The suspension was then injected through a sharp-ended needle with an inner diameter of 300 μm into the immiscible liquid paraffin stream under laminar flow maintained at 37°C. The resultant droplets of agarose solution in the liquid paraffin were collected in a tube and subsequently cooled in an ice bath for 10 min. We collected the gelled agarose microparticles into an aqueous phase by centrifugation after adding saline buffer solution. The viability of mouse insulinoma (MIN-6) cells enclosed in the resultant agarose microparticles about 80 μm in diameter was 89.2% [45].

We indirectly evaluated growth profiles of cells encapsulated in agarose microparticles by measuring the transition of mitochondrial activity of enclosed cells per microparticle from the increase in water-soluble formazan dye generated by the dehydrogenase within intact mitochondria in living cells using a colorimetric assay kit (Cell Counting kit-8, Dojindo, Kumamoto, Japan). As typically shown for the Crandall Reese feline kidney (CRFK) cells encapsulated in agarose microparticles of about 100 μm in diameter, the microparticle-based mitochondrial activity increased during the first week and achieved more than twice the initial (day 1) value (Fig. **7**) [50]. Subsequently, the microparticle-based activity gradually decreased during the culturing period which followed. Although the mechanism for the decrease in mitochondrial activity after 1 week of encapsulation is still unclear, this tendency for viability to increase during the early cultivation period, followed by a subsequent gradual decrease is not specific to the agarose microparticles obtained using our method. It is in agreement with the result reported for several kinds of mammalian cells enclosed in microparticles made from alginate-agarose composites with diameters of 350 to 450 μm [64]. One possible explanation for the suppression of the cellular growth is the existence of limited space for cell proliferation and the solid stress induced by the surrounding agarose gel. Cell proliferation is only possible in the small space that was originally filled with individual cells at the actual time of agarose gelation. In fact, almost all the enclosed cells maintained their initial appearance in agarose microparticles (Fig. **8**) [51]. Regarding the effect of solid stress on the growth of enclosed cells, it was reported that the cloning efficiency of tumor cells enclosed in 1.8% agarose gel was only 5% despite the fact that in a 1.0% gel it was more than 90% [55]. Therefore, decreasing the solid stress induced by the surrounding agarose gel may prolong the therapeutic functional period of cell-enclosing microparticles as a result of cell growth within them. However, the risk of leakage of enclosed cells into the surrounding environment should also be considered from a safety point of view when implanting *in vivo*. In the case of transplanting a proliferative cell line *in vivo*, suppression of the excess proliferation of enclosed cells is vital to avoid the risk of tumorigenesis [21].

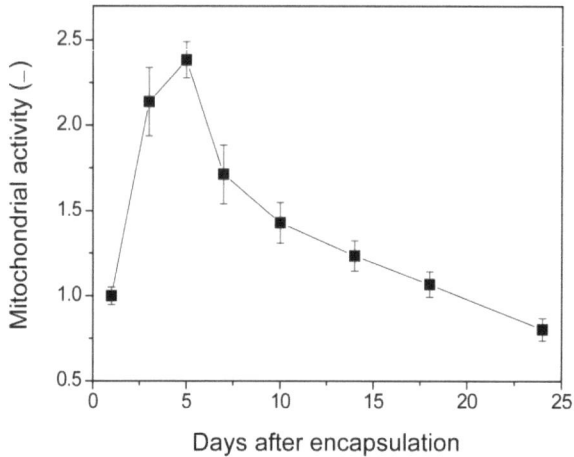

Figure 7: Mitochondrial activity of enclosed cells in subsieve-size agarose capsules prepared through the flow focusing process. Bars: SDs. Mitochondrial activity is a dimensionless value normalized against the value measured 1 day after encapsulation. (Reproduced with permission from Sakai *et al.* Biochem Eng J [50] @2006 Elsevier).

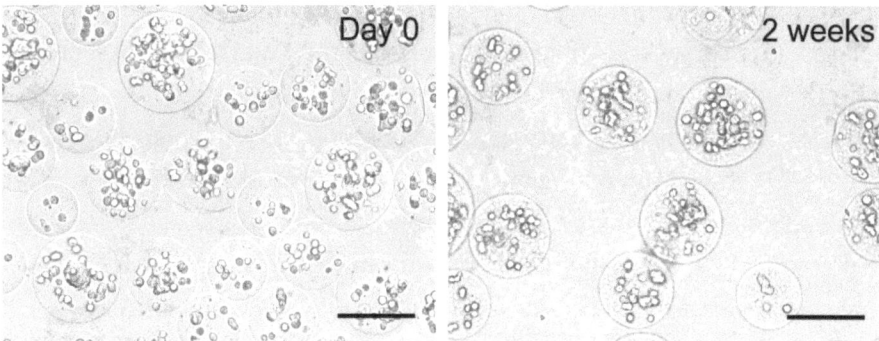

Figure 8: Appearances of cells enclosed in agarose microparticles at days 0, 2 weeks after encapsulation. Bars: 150 μm.

3.2. Alginate-Ph Microparticles

Alginates are an interesting family of polysaccharides that have been studied for a wide variety of biomedical applications [4, 65-69]. They are abundant in nature and are found as structural components in marine brown algae and as capsular polysaccharides in some soil bacteria. There are issues to be solved for practical clinical applications such as difficulties of purification resulting in immunogenicity when implanted [70] and challenges with freezing/thawing. Despite this they have been the most frequently used material for cell-encapsulation since the first report in the 1980s [1]. Alginates have two attractive characteristics as a material for cell-enclosing vehicles. One is that the aqueous sodium-alginate solution is gellable in the presence of divalent cations under very mild conditions for mammalian cells. The other attractive point is that polyelectrolyte layers can be prepared on the resultant alginate microparticles by soaking them in an aqueous solution containing cationic polymers such as poly-L-lysine and chitosan for enhancement of mechanical stability and for controlling molecular exchangeability [71-74]. A well-known drawback of ionically cross-linked Ca-alginate gels obtained from native sodium-alginate is their limited mechanical stability under physiological conditions [75]. This low stability results from the exchange of cross-linking calcium ions with non-gel-inducing sodium ions. We originally developed alginate with hydroxyl phenol moieties in the polymer side chains (Alg-Ph) to solve this problem by forming covalent cross-linking between alginate molecules [76]. Because of the existence of hydroxyl phenol moieties, an aqueous solution of the alginate derivative is gellable through a horseradish peroxidase (HRP) catalyzed oxidative reaction using H_2O_2, resulting in C-C and C-O coupling of phenols (Fig. **9**) [77-79]. Less than 5% of hydroxyl phenol moieties incorporated on the original carboxyl groups of alginate and the enzymatic cross-linking formation between these moieties was effective for enhancing the stability of the resultant gel [76, 80]. Because more than 90% of the original carboxyl groups remain, the aqueous solution is gellable through not only the peroxidase catalyzed reaction but also the conventional gelation process in the presence of multivalent cations. We applied Alg-Ph to the production of cell-enclosing microparticles using droplet breakup in a water-immiscible liquid stream with laminar flow.

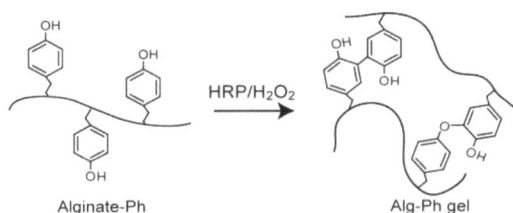

Figure 9: Gelation scheme for the gelation of Alg-Ph by HRP-catalyzed oxidative coupling of phenols.

A problem at the starting point of the study was how to supply the H_2O_2 necessary for the HRP-catalyzed cross-linking reaction. One option was to inject a mixture of Alg-Ph, HRP and H_2O_2 into the co-flowing liquid paraffin stream. However, this was not practical for continuous production of cell-enclosing microparticles because of gelation of the mixture in the syringe before or during extrusion from the needle. From the view point of continuous production, we developed a method for supplying H_2O_2 from the liquid paraffin to the droplets of Alg-Ph solution containing HRP [53]. Although liquid paraffin is a water-immiscible liquid, usually such a water-immiscible liquid can dissolve a small quantity of water. We vigorously stirred an aqueous H_2O_2 solution (31%) with liquid paraffin at a volume ratio of 5: 1000. We then centrifuged the solution to separate the liquid paraffin and non-dissolved aqueous H_2O_2 solution. Using the resultant liquid paraffin as an ambient liquid, partially gelated Alg-Ph microparticles in liquid paraffin were collected in a plastic tube. After 10 min of standing to allow for further progress of the HRP-catalyzed cross-linking reaction, Alg-Ph microparticles were collected through centrifugation, the same as for agarose microparticles. As shown in Fig. **10**, the resultant Alg-Ph microparticles had high sphericity.

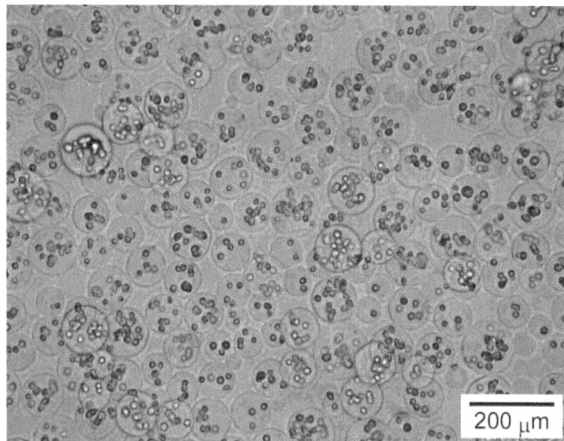

Figure 10: Micrograph of CRFK cell-enclosing Alg-Ph capsules of diameter 84.8 ± 13 µm. (Reproduced with permission from Sakai *et al.* Biomacromolecules [53]@2007 American Chemical Society).

One of the concerns for this HRP-catalyzed microparticle production process would be the potential damage of mammalian cells resulting from exposure to

H_2O_2 because the cytotoxicity of H_2O_2 is well-known. However, we could not find this in studies using CRFK cells [53]. The viability of cells retrieved from 100 μm Alg-Ph microparticles after 30 min of encapsulation by degrading the Alg-Ph gel using alginate lyase was more than 90%, almost the same as the viability detected for cells enclosed in non-gelled droplets of sodium-alginate solution [46]. In addition, cells retrieved from Alg-Ph microparticles showed the same growth profile as cells seeded using a general subculture protocol after showing the same adhesion rate at 4 hours after seeding (Fig. **11**).

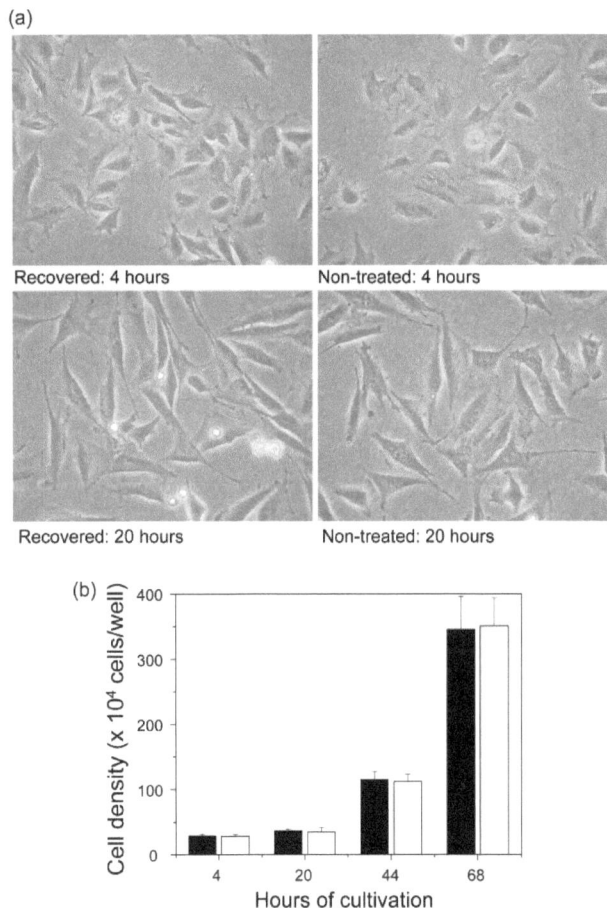

Figure 11: (a) Micrographs of CRFK cells cultured on cell culture dishes 60 μm in diameter at 4 and 20 hours after seeding. Recovered: cells seeded after being recovered from Alg-Ph capsules by degradation using alginate lyase. Non-treated: cells seeded using a general subculture protocol. Cells were seeded at 3.0×10^5 viable cells/well. (b) Proliferation profiles of CRFK cells on tissue culture dishes. Columns indicate mean densities of (black) recovered cells and (white) non-treated

cells. Bars: SDs. (Reproduced with permission, from Sakai *et al.* Biomacromolecules [53]@ 2007 American Chemical Society).

We believe this promising result was induced by the gradual and minor penetration of H_2O_2 from the liquid paraffin into the droplets containing Alg-Ph and HRP, and the immediate consumption of the penetrated H_2O_2 by the HRP-catalyzed reaction. In contrast to cells enclosed in agarose microparticles, microparticle-based mitochondrial activity of cells enclosed in Alg-Ph microparticles gradually increased with increasing cultivation time and achieved about a 10-times higher value after 2 months of encapsulation compared with the value at day 1. The growth of cells in Alg-Ph microparticles was clearly recognized from the increase in the space occupied by the cells in the microparticles (Fig. **12**). The majority of the microparticles contained cellular clumps 20-70 μm in diameter after 65 days of encapsulation.

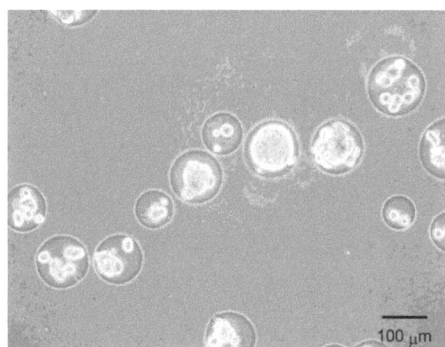

Figure 12: Micrograph of CRFK cell-enclosing Alg-Ph microparticles after 65 days of encapsulation. (Reproduced with permission, from Sakai *et al.* Biomacromolecules [53]@ 2007 American Chemical Society).

3.3. Agarose Microcapsules

The vehicles described above are microparticles. In these microparticles, proliferation of enclosed cells is constrained by microscopic stresses arising from the surrounding gel [55, 81]. For the growth of enclosed cells, microcapsules with a hollow core, *i.e.* in which cells are surrounded by liquid, are preferable [82-84]. Not only are the cells in this case free from the solid stress but also higher diffusivities of oxygen, nutrients and metabolites in the liquid than in the gel are considered to explain the higher cellular growth observed in liquid-core microcapsules [73]. To date, the majority of cell-enclosing microcapsules have been made from alginate and cationic polymers [1, 85, 86]. They are prepared by sequentially immersing cell-enclosing calcium-alginate microparticles in a cationic polymer aqueous solution, an anionic polymer solution for the formation of a polyelectrolyte complex microcapsule membrane layer and finally a calcium-chelating reagent solution to liquefy the core calcium-alginate gel [3]. A drawback of the process, including the penetration of counter-charged polymers, is that cells entrapped very close to the surface of the calcium-alginate microparticles are incorporated into the resultant polyelectrolyte complex layer and some cells are exposed on the surface [87]. Increasing the cell content in the original calcium-alginate microparticles increases the risks of cellular leakage to the surrounding environment, consequent decreases in the mechanical stability and deterioration of the immuno-isolation properties of the polyelectrolyte complex layer [88].

We developed a novel technique for obtaining hollow-core microcapsules with the microcapsule membrane free of cells using the droplet breakup technique in a water-immiscible liquid stream with laminar flow [87]. The microcapsules are prepared from Alg-Ph and agarose. First, cell-enclosing Alg-Ph microparticles about 150 μm in diameter are prepared through the HRP-catalyzed cross linking reaction method described above. The Alg-Ph microparticles are then suspended in a 50-times larger volume of aqueous agarose solution. The agarose solution is extruded into the co-flowing liquid paraffin under a flow rate by which agarose microparticles less than 50 μm are obtained. The size distribution of the resultant agarose microparticles showed two clear, non-overlapping peaks, about 50 μm and about 200 μm in diameter (Fig. **13**). All of the 200 μm microparticles contained Alg-Ph microparticles about 150 μm in diameter. The non-overlapping size distribution indicates that agarose microparticles enclosing Alg-Ph microparticles are easily separated using a filter with an appropriate pore size. Such a simple separation technique for removing vehicles that do not contain cells is attractive for cell therapy applications because there is a limit to the volume of cell-enclosing vehicles that can be implanted. We prepared the hollow-core structure by degrading the core Alg-Ph microparticles using alginate lyase. The degradation step consists simply of soaking the resultant microparticles in a medium containing alginate lyase for 1 hr. An attractive feature of this technique is that the size of the hollow core can easily be defined by the diameter of the Alg-Ph microparticles used as the template.

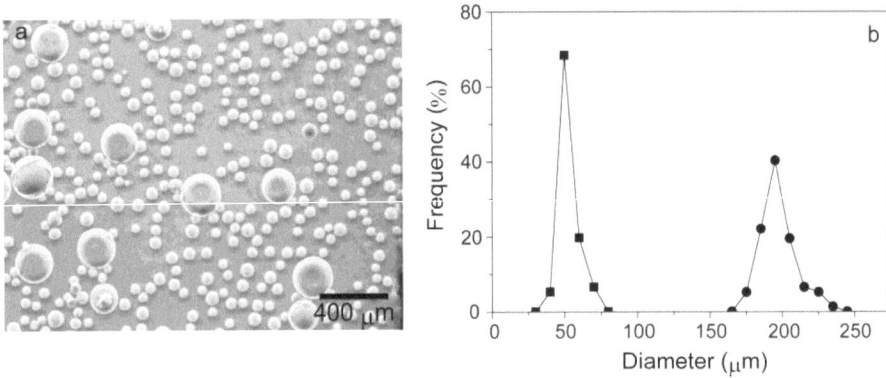

Figure 13: (a) Agarose microparticles enclosing (large particles) or not enclosing (small particles) a single alginate microparticle of ca. 150 μm in diameter. (b) Size distribution of agarose microparticles enclosing (●) or not enclosing (■) a single alginate microparticle. (Reproduced with permission from Sakai *et al.* Biotechnol Bioeng [87] @2008 Wiley Periodicals, Inc.).

We enclosed CRFK cells in agarose microcapsules with hollow cores of about 150 μm in diameter and compared their growth profiles with those of cells enclosed in Alg-Ph microparticles by the indirect method based on mitochondrial activity. The mitochondrial activity per vehicle continued to increase until 53 days after encapsulation and reached an approximately 50-fold higher value relative to the value measured on the day after encapsulation. The growth profile was much faster than that of the cells enclosed in Alg-Ph microparticles (Fig. **14**).

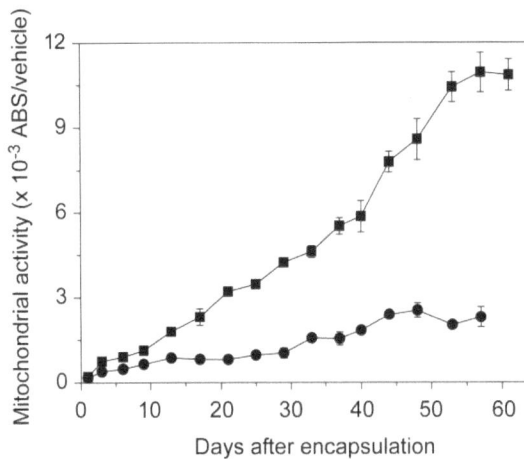

Figure 14: Transition of mitochondrial activities of CRFK cells enclosed in (■) agarose microcapsules with a hollow core of ca. 150 μm in diameter and (●) alginate microparticles used as a template for the hollow cores of agarose microcapsules. Bars: SDs. (Reproduced with permission from Sakai *et al.* Biotechnol Bioeng [87] @2008 Wiley Periodicals, Inc.).

This result clearly indicates the effectiveness of the hollow-core structure developed using Alg-Ph microparticles as templates for enhancing growth of enclosed cells. In addition, suppression of cellular growth in the agarose microcapsules was indicated by the unchanged mitochondrial activity from day 53 to day 60. This growth suppression is explained by the existence of the agarose microcapsule membrane [87]. As shown (Fig. **15**), the hollow cores were completely filled by cells by 45 days of encapsulation.

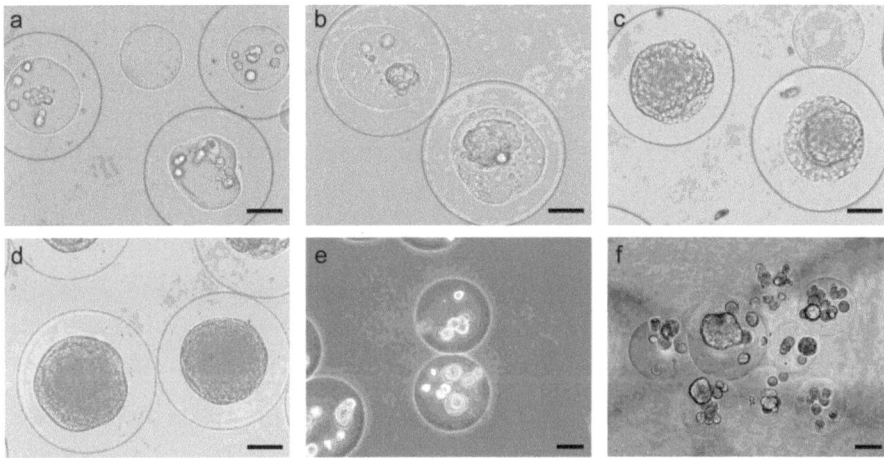

Figure 15: Micrographs of CRFK cells enclosed in (a-d) agarose microcapsules and (e, f) alginate microparticles (a, e) just after encapsulation, on (b) day 14, (c) day 30, (d) day 45, and (f) day 49. Bars: 50 μm. (Reproduced with permission from Sakai *et al.* Biotechnol Bioeng [87]@2008 Wiley Periodicals, Inc.).

4. POSSIBILITYY FOR CELL THERAPY

We studied the potential for cell therapy using the above mentioned agarose microparticles and agarose microcapsules. We examined this potential for localized chemotherapy by providing an alternative site for the activation of a prodrug, ifosfamide, which normally occurs in the liver, inside or near tumors. Ifosfamide is a prodrug that is specifically metabolized in the liver into two major active compounds, phosphoramide mustard and acrolein, by cytochrome P450 2B1 (CYP2B1) [89]. Because of the very short half-life of the activated compounds in plasma [90], ifosfamide has to be given in relatively high doses, despite the occurrence of severe side effects associated with such doses, such as leucopenia with granulocytopenia. Lohr *et al.,* [91] reported a method for reducing the side effects without lowering response rates by establishing a second site of enzyme conversion near or inside the tumor by bringing cells transfected to express CYP2B1 close to the tumor. The effectiveness of this approach was shown in a clinical trial by placing microcapsules of conventional size enclosing the cells in an artery near the tumor by microcatheter [92, 93].

We enclosed CRFK cells genetically engineered to express the liver active enzyme CYP2B1 [91] in agarose microparticles about 100 μm in diameter and agarose microcapsules about 150 μm in diameter with hollow cores about 100 μm in diameter. These vehicles were implanted using a 26-gauge needle after suspension in saline to nude mice bearing pre-established tumors established by subcutaneously transplanting a human squamous carcinoma cell line. The small sizes of our vehicles allowed the use of such a small needle for implantation. For both vehicles, microparticles and microcapsules, significant regression of tumors was observed compared with those implanted with empty vehicles [94, 95] (Fig. **16**). In this chapter we have not discussed preferred structures of cell-enclosing vehicles (microparticles or microcapsules) for cell therapy, because we think this strongly depends on the characteristics of the enclosed cells and the kind of disease. Important findings were that the enclosed cells functioned in both our agarose microparticles and agarose microcapsules *in vivo*.

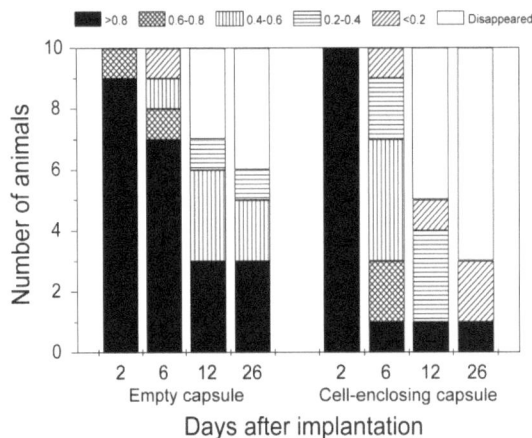

Figure 16: Preformed tumor size changes of the recipients transplanted empty and CYP2B1 cells-enclosing subsieve-size agarose capsules. Ten nude mice each were used as recipients of empty and cell-enclosing capsules. Tumor size just before capsule implantation was set to 1 and each block represents the proportional size of the original tumor. (Reproduced with permission from Sakai *et al.* Mol Cancer Ther [94] @2005 American Association for Cancer Research).

5. CONCLUSION

In this chapter, we described methods for the production of cell-enclosing microparticles and microcapsules of about 100-200 μm in diameter, which are smaller than conventional ones (300-1,000 μm in diameter) using droplet breakup in a water-immiscible liquid stream with laminar flow. Features of the method are that droplets with diameters even less than 100 μm can be prepared using a needle several hundred micrometers in diameter and the droplet breakup process is mild enough for mammalian cells. We introduced two microparticles and one microcapsule. The microparticles were prepared through a thermal gelation process using agarose and an HRP-catalyzed gelation process using Alg-Ph. The microcapsule was prepared by covering the Alg-Ph microparticles with an agarose gel layer and subsequently degrading the Alg-Ph microparticle enzymatically. Studies for cell therapy using these small vehicles are still at an early stage with respect to practical applications. However, we believe the small vehicles prepared using the droplet breakup method will become useful devices for cell therapy.

ACKNOWLEDGEMENT

None declared.

CONFLICT OF INTEREST

The author(s) confirm that this chapter content has no conflict of interest.

REFERENCES

[1]   Lim F, Sun AM. Microencapsulated islets as bioartificial endocrine pancreas. Science 1980; 210: 908-10.
[2]   Rihova B. Immunocompatibility and biocompatibility of cell delivery systems. Adv Drug Deliv Rev 2000; 42: 65-80.
[3]   Uludag H, de Vos P, Tresco PA. Technology of mammalian cell encapsulation. Adv Drug Deliv Rev 2000; 42: 29-64.
[4]   Zimmermann H, Zimmermann D, Reuss R, Feilen PJ, Manz B, Katsen A *et al.* Towards a medically approved technology for alginate-based microcapsules allowing long-term immunoisolated transplantation. J Mater Sci Mater Med 2005; 16: 491-501.
[5]   Murua A, Portero A, Orive G, Hernandez RM, de Castro M, Pedraz JL. Cell microencapsulation technology: towards clinical application. J Control Release 2008; 132: 76-83.

[6]   Bartkowiak A, Hunkeler D. New microcapsules based on oligoelectrolyte complexation. Ann N Y Acad Sci 1999; 875: 36-45.

[7]   Yoshioka T, Hirano R, Shioya T, Kako M. Encapsulation of mammalian cell with chitosan-CMC capsule. Biotechnol Bioeng 1990; 35: 66-72.

[8]   Zhang W J, Marx S -K, Laue Ch, Hyder A, Juergensen A, Bickel M *et al.* HOE 077 reduces fibrotic overgrowth around the barium alginate microcapsule. Transplant Proc 2000; 32: 206-9.

[9]   Lu MZ, Lan HL, Wang FF, Chang SJ, Wang YJ. Cell encapsulation with alginate and alpha-phenoxycinnamylidene-acetylated poly(allylamine). Biotechnol Bioeng 2000; 70: 479-83.

[10]   Wang YJ. Development of new polycations for cell encapsulation with alginate. Mater Sci Eng C 2000; 13: 59-63.

[11]   Dautzenberg H, Schuldt U, Grasnick G, Karle P, Muller P, Lohr M *et al.* Development of cellulose sulfate-based polyelectrolyte complex microcapsules for medical applications. Ann N Y Acad Sci 1999; 875: 46-63.

[12]   Sakai S, Ono T, Ijima H, Kawakami K. Synthesis and transport characterization of alginate/aminopropyl-silicate/alginate microcapsule: application to bioartificial pancreas. Biomaterials 2001; 22: 2827-34.

[13]   Canaple L, Rehor A, Hunkeler D. Improving cell encapsulation through size control. J Biomater Sci Polym Ed 2002; 13: 783-96.

[14]   Kim SK, Yu SH, Son JH, Hübner H, Buchholz R. Calculations on O_2 transfer in capsules with animal cells for the determination of maximum capsule size without O_2 limitation. Biotechnol Lett 1998; 20: 549-52.

[15]   Chicheportiche D, Reach G. *In vitro* kinetics of insulin release by microencapsulated rat islets: effect of the size of the microcapsules. Diabetologia 1988; 31: 54-7.

[16]   Robitaille R, Pariseau J-F, Leblong FA, Lamoureux M, Lepage Y, Halle J-P. Studies on small (<350 μm) alginate-poly-L-lysine microcapsules. III. Biocompatibility of smaller *vs.* standard microcapsules. J Biomed Mater Res 1999; 44: 116-20.

[17]   Strand BL, Gasero O, Kulseng B, Espevik T, Skjak-Braek G. Alginate-polylysine-alginate microcapsules: effect of size reduction on capsule properties. J Microencapsul 2002; 19: 615-30.

[18]   de Vos P, De Haan B, Pater J, Van Schilfgaarde R. Association between capsule diameter, adequacy of encapsulation, and survival of microencapsulated rat islet allografts. Transplantation 1996; 62: 893-9.

[19]   Chang TM. Therapeutic applications of polymeric artificial cells. Nat Rev Drug Discov 2005; 4: 221-35.

[20]   Hauser O, Prieschl Grassauer E, Salmons B. Encapsulated, genetically modified cells producing *in vivo* therapeutics. Curr Opin Mol Ther 2004; 6: 412-20.

[21]   Chang PL, Van Raamsdonk JM, Hortelano G, Barsoum SC, MacDonald NC, Stockley TL. The *in vivo* delivery of heterologous proteins by microencapsulated recombinant cells. Trends Biotechnol 1999; 17: 78-83.

[22]   Joki T, Machluf M, Atala A, Zhu JH, Seyfried NT, Dunn IF *et al.* Continuous release of endostatin from microencapsulated engineered cells for tumor therapy. Nat Biotechnol 2001; 19: 35-9.

[23]   Muller P, Jesnowski R, Karle P, Renz R, Saller R, Stein H *et al.* Injection of encapsulated cells producing an ifosfamide-activating cytochrome P450 for targeted chemotherapy to pancreatic tumors. Ann N Y Acad Sci 1999; 880: 337-51.

[24]   Read TA, Sorensen DR, Mahesparan R, Enger PO, Timpl R, Olsen BR *et al.* Local endostatin treatment of gliomas administered by microencapsulated producer cells. Nat Biotechnol 2001; 19: 29-34.

[25]   Chicheportiche D, Reach G. *In vitro* kinetics of insulin release by microencapsulated rat islets: effect of the size of the microcapsules. Diabetologia 1988; 31: 54-7.

[26]   Schrezenmeir J, Gero L, Solhdju M, Kirchgessner J, Laue C, Beyer J *et al.* Relation between secretory function and oxygen supply in isolated islet organs. Transplant Proc 1994; 26: 809-13.

[27]   Leblond FA, Simard G, Henley N, Rocheleau B, Huet PM, Halle JP. Studies on smaller (approximately 315 μm) microcapsules: IV. Feasibility and safety of intrahepatic implantations of small alginate poly-L-lysine microcapsules. Cell Transplant 1999; 8: 327-37.

[28]   Ross CJ, Chang PL. Development of small alginate microcapsules for recombinant gene product delivery to the rodent brain. J Biomater Sci Polym Ed 2002; 13: 953-62.

[29]   Sugiura S, Oda T, Aoyagi Y, Matsuo R, Enomoto T, Matsumoto K *et al.* Microfabricated airflow nozzle for microencapsulation of living cells into 150 micrometer microcapsules. Biomed Microdevices 2007; 9: 91-9.

[30]   Sugiura S, Oda T, Izumida Y, Aoyagi Y, Satake M, Ochiai A *et al.* Size control of calcium alginate beads containing living cells using micro-nozzle array. Biomaterials 2005; 26: 3327-31.

[31]   Choi CH, Jung JH, Rhee YW, Kim DP, Shim SE, Lee CS. Generation of monodisperse alginate microbeads and *in situ* encapsulation of cell in microfluidic device. Biomed Microdevices 2007; 9: 855-62.

[32]   Sparks RE, Salemme RM, Meier PM, Litt MH, Lindan O. Removal of waste metabolites in uremia by microencapsulated reactants. Trans Amer Soc Artif Int Organs 1969; 15: 353-9.

[33]   Eiselt P, Yeh J, Latvala RK, Shea LD, Mooney DJ. Porous carriers for biomedical applications based on alginate hydrogels. Biomaterials 2000; 21: 1921-7.

[34]   Sakai S, Ono T, Ijima H, Kawakami K. Control of molecular weight cut-off for immunoisolation by multilayering glycol chitosan-alginate polyion complex on alginate-based microcapsule. J Microencapsul 2000; 17: 691-9.

[35]   Leung A, Ramaswamy Y, Munro P, Lawrie G, Nielsen L, Trau M. Emulsion strategies in the microencapsulation of cells: pathways to thin coherent membranes. Biotechnol Bioeng 2005; 92: 45-53.

[36]   Pajic-Lijakovic I, Bugarski D, Plavsic M, Bugarski B. Influence of microenvironmental conditions on hybridoma cell growth inside the alginate-poly-L-lysine microcapsule. Process Biochem 2007; 42: 167-74.

[37]   Chang PL, Hortelano G, Tse M, Awrey DE. Growth of recombinant fibroblasts in alginate microcapsules. Biotechnol Bioeng 1994; 43: 925-33.

[38]   Zhang Y, Wang W, Zhou J, Yu W, Zhang X, Guo X *et al.* Tumor anti-angiogenic gene therapy with microencapsulated recombinant CHO cells. Ann Biomed Eng 2007; 35: 605-14.

[39]   Wolters GH, Fritschy WM, Gerrits D, van Schilfgaarde R. A versatile alginate droplet generator applicable for microencapsulation of pancreatic islets. J Appl Biomater 1992; 3: 281-6.

[40]   Ganan-Calvo AM. Generation of steady liquid microthreads and micron-sized monodisperse sprays in gas streams. Phys Rev Lett 1998; 80: 285-8.

[41] Nir R, Lamed R, Gueta L, Sahar E. Single-cell entrapment and microcolony development within uniform microspheres amenable to flow cytometry. Appl Environ Microb 1990; 56: 2870-5.

[42] Zhang DF, Stone HA. Drop formation in viscous flows at a vertical capillary tube. Phys Fluids 1997; 9: 2234-42.

[43] Lim ST, Martin GP, Berry DJ, Brown MB. Preparation and evaluation of the *in vitro* drug release properties and mucoadhesion of novel microspheres of hyaluronic acid and chitosan. J Control Release 2000; 66: 281-92.

[44] Ribeiro AJ, Neufeld RJ, Arnaud P, Chaumeil JC. Microencapsulation of lipophilic drugs in chitosan-coated alginate microspheres. Int J Pharm 1999; 187: 115-23.

[45] Sakai S, Kawabata K, Ono T, Ijima H, Kawakami K. Development of mammalian cell-enclosing subsieve-size agarose capsules (<100 μm) for cell therapy. Biomaterials 2005; 26: 4786-92.

[46] Sakai S, Kawabata K, Ono T, Ijima H, Kawakami K. Preparation of mammalian cell-enclosing subsieve-sized capsules (<100 μm) in a coflowing stream. Biotechnol Bioeng 2004; 86: 168-73.

[47] Sakai S, Kawabata K, Ono T, Ijima H, Kawakami K. Higher viscous solution induces smaller droplets for cell-enclosing capsules in a co-flowing stream. Biotechnol Prog 2005; 21: 994-7.

[48] Cramer C, Fischer P, Windhab EJ. Drop formation in a co-flowing ambient fluid. Chem Eng Sci 2004; 59: 3045-58.

[49] Rayleigh JWS. On the stability of jets. Proc Lond Math Soc 1878; 10: 4-11.

[50] Sakai S, Hashimoto I, Kawakami K. Usefulness of flow focusing technology for producing subsieve-size cell enclosing capsules: Application for agarose capsules production. Biochem Eng J 2006; 30: 218-21.

[51] Sakai S, Hashimoto I, Kawakami K. Agarose-gelatin conjugate for adherent cell-enclosing capsules. Biotechnol Lett 2007; 29: 731-5.

[52] Sakai S, Hashimoto I, Kawakami K. Development of alginate-agarose subsieve-size capsules for subsequent modification with a polyelectrolyte complex membrane. Biochem Eng J 2006; 30: 76-81.

[53] Sakai S, Hashimoto I, Ogushi Y, Kawakami K. Peroxidase-catalyzed cell-encapsulation in subsieve-size capsules of alginate with phenol moieties in water-immiscible fluid dissolving H_2O_2. Biomacromolecules 2007; 8: 2622-6.

[54] Sakai S, Ito S, Ogushi Y, Kawakami K. Feasibility of carboxymethylcellulose with phenol moieties as a material for mammalian cell-enclosing subsieve-size capsules. Cellulose 2008; 15: 723-9.

[55] Helmlinger G, Netti PA, Lichtenbeld HC, Melder RJ, Jain RK. Solid stress inhibits the growth of multicellular tumor spheroids. Nat Biotechnol 1997; 15: 778-83.

[56] Bougault C, Paumier A, Aubert Foucher E, Mallein Gerin F. Molecular analysis of chondrocytes cultured in agarose in response to dynamic compression. BMC Biotechnol 2008; 8: 71.

[57] Bougault C, Paumier A, Aubert Foucher E, Mallein Gerin F. Investigating conversion of mechanical force into biochemical signaling in three-dimensional chondrocyte cultures. Nat Protoc 2009; 4: 928-38.

[58] Sasazaki Y, Seedhom BB, Shore R. Morphology of the bovine chondrocyte and of its cytoskeleton in isolation and *in situ*: are chondrocytes ubiquitously paired through the entire layer of articular cartilage?. Rheumatology (Oxford) 2008; 47: 1641-6.

[59] Rahfoth B, Weisser J, Sternkopf F, Aigner T, von der Mark K, Brauer R. Transplantation of allograft chondrocytes embedded in agarose gel into cartilage defects of rabbits. Osteoarthr Cartilage 1998; 6: 50-65.

[60] Dimicco MA, Kisiday JD, Gong H, Grodzinsky AJ. Structure of pericellular matrix around agarose-embedded chondrocytes. Osteoarthritis Cartilage 2007; 15: 1207-16.

[61] Tashiro H, Iwata H, Warnock GL, Ikada Y, Tsuji T. Viability studies of agarose microencapsulation islets of Langerhans from dogs. Transplant Proc 1998; 30: 490.

[62] Tun T, Inoue K, Hayashi H, Aung T, Gu Y-J, Doi R *et al.* A newly developed three-layer agarose microcapsule for a promising biohybrid artificial pancreas: Rat to mouse xenotransplantation. Cell Transplant 1996; 5: S59-63.

[63] Iwata H, Murakami Y, Ikada Y. Control of complement activities for immunoisolation. Ann N Y Acad Sci 1999; 875: 7-23.

[64] Orive G, Hernandez RM, Gascon AR, Igartua M, Pedraz JL. Survival of different cell lines in alginate-agarose microcapsules. Eur J Pharm Sci 2003; 18: 23-30.

[65] Gutowska A, Jeong B, Jasionowski M. Injectable gels for tissue engineering. Anat Rec 2001; 263: 342-9.

[66] Caterson EJ, Li WJ, Nesti LJ, Albert T, Danielson K, Tuan RS. Polymer/alginate amalgam for cartilage-tissue engineering. Ann N Y Acad Sci 2002; 961: 134-8.

[67] Chung TW, Yang J, Akaike T, Cho KY, Nah JW, Kim SI *et al.* Preparation of alginate/galactosylated chitosan scaffold for hepatocyte attachment. Biomaterials 2002; 23: 2827-34.

[68] Weber M, Steinert A, Jork A, Dimmler A, Thurmer F, Schutze N *et al.* Formation of cartilage matrix proteins by BMP-transfected murine mesenchymal stem cells encapsulated in a novel class of alginates. Biomaterials 2002; 23: 2003-13.

[69] Marijnissen WJ, van Osch GJ, Aigner J, van der Veen SW, Hollander AP, Verwoerd Verhoef HL *et al.* Alginate as a chondrocyte-delivery substance in combination with a non-woven scaffold for cartilage tissue engineering. Biomaterials 2002; 23: 1511-7.

[70] Ménard M, Dusseault J, Langlois G, Baille WE, Tam SK, Yahia L *et al.* Role of protein contaminants in the immunogenicity of alginates. J Biomed Mater Res B Appl Biomater. 2010; 93:333-40.

[71] Goosen MFA, O'Shea GM, Gharapetian HM, Chou S, Sun AM. Optimization of microencapsulation parameters: Semipermeable microcapsules as a bioartificial pancreas. Biotechnol Bioeng 1985; 27: 146-50.

[72] Goosen MFA, King GA, McKnight CA, Marcotte N. Animal cell culture engineering using alginate polycation microcapsules of controlled membrane molecular weight cut-off. J Membr Sci 1989; 41: 323-43.

[73] Thu B, Bruheim P, Espevik T, Smidsrod O, Soon-Shiong P, Skjak-Braek G. Alginate polycation microcapsules.2. Some functional properties. Biomaterials 1996; 17: 1069-79.

[74] Thu B, Bruheim P, Espevik T, Smidsrod O, Soon-Shiong P, Skjak-Braek G. Alginate polycation microcapsules.1. Interaction between alginate and polycation. Biomaterials 1996; 17: 1031-40.

[75] Smidsrod O, Skjak-Braek G. Alginate as immobilization matrix for cells. Trends Biotechnol 1990; 8: 71-8.

[76] Sakai S, Kawakami K. Synthesis and characterization of both ionically and enzymatically crosslinkable alginate. Acta Biomater 2007; 3: 495-501.

[77]   Kurisawa M, Chung JE, Yang YY, Gao SJ, Uyama H. Injectable biodegradable hydrogels composed of hyaluronic acid-tyramine conjugates for drug delivery and tissue engineering. Chem Comm 2005; 34: 4312-4.

[78]   Fukuda T, Uyama H, Kobayashi S. Polymerization of polyfunctional macromolecules: synthesis of a new class of high molecular weight poly(amino acid)s by oxidative coupling of phenol-containing precursor polymers. Biomacromolecules 2004; 5: 977-83.

[79]   Kobayashi S, Uyama H, Kimura S. Enzymatic Polymerization. Chem Rev 2001; 101: 3793-818.

[80]   Sakai S, Kawakami K. Both Ionically and enzymatically crosslinkable alginate-tyramine conjugate as materials for cell encapsulation. J Biomed Mater Res 2008; 85A: 345-51.

[81]   Cadic C, Dupuy B, Pianet I, Merle M, Margerin C, Bezian JH. *In vitro* culture of hybridoma cells in agarose beads producing antibody secretion for 2 weeks. Biotechnol Bioeng 1992; 39: 108-12.

[82]   Constantinidis I, Rask I, Long RC Jr, Sambanis A. Effects of alginate composition on the metabolic, secretory, and growth characteristics of entrapped beta TC3 mouse insulinoma cells. Biomaterials 1999; 20: 2019-27.

[83]   Garfinkel MR, Harland RC, Opara EC. Optimization of the microencapsulated islets for transplantation. J Surg Res 1998; 76: 7-10.

[84]   Wang X, Wang W, Ma J, Guo X, Yu X, Ma X. Proliferation and differentiation of mouse embryonic stem cells in APA microcapsule: A model for studying the interaction between stem cells and their niche. Biotechnol Prog 2006; 22: 791-800.

[85]   Calafiore R, Basta G, Luca G, Boselli C, Bufalari A, Giustozzi GA *et al.* Alginate/polyaminoacides coherent microcapsules for pancreatic islet graft immunoisolation in diabetic recipients. Ann N Y Acad Sci 1997; 831: 313-22.

[86]   Orive G, Tam SK, Pedraz JL, Halle JP. Biocompatibility of biomaterials for cell microencapsulation. Biomaterials 2006; 27: 3691-700.

[87]   Sakai S, Hashimoto I, Kawakami K. Production of cell-enclosing hollow-core agarose microcapsules *via* jetting in water-immiscible liquid paraffin and formation of embryoid body-like spherical tissues from mouse ES cells enclosed within these microcapsules. Biotechnol Bioeng 2008; 99: 235-43.

[88]   Wong H, Chang TM. A novel two step procedure for immobilizing living cells in microcapsules for improving xenograft survival. Biomater Artif Cells Immobilization Biotechnol 1991; 19: 687-97.

[89]   Dirven HA, Megens L, Oudshoorn MJ, Dingemanse MA, van Ommen B, van Bladeren PJ. Glutathione conjugation of the cytostatic drug ifosfamide and the role of human glutathione S-transferases. Chem Res Toxicol 1995; 8: 979-86.

[90]   Kurowski V, Wagner T. Comparative pharmacokinetics of ifosfamide, 4-hydroxyifosfamide, chloroacetaldehyde, and 2- and 3-dechloroethylifosfamide in patients on fractionated intravenous ifosfamide therapy. Cancer Chemother Pharmacol 1993; 33: 36-42.

[91]   Lohr M, Muller P, Karle P, Stange J, Mitzner S, Jesnowski R *et al.* Targeted chemotherapy by intratumour injection of encapsulated cells engineered to produce CYP2B1, an ifosfamide activating cytochrome P450. Gene Ther 1998; 5: 1070-8.

[92]   Lohr M, Kroger JC, Hoffmeyer A, Freund M, Hain J, Holle A *et al.* Safety, feasibility and clinical benefit of localized chemotherapy using microencapsulated cells for inoperable pancreatic carcinoma in a phase I/II trial. Cancer Therapy 2003; 1: 121-31.

[93]   Lohr M, Hoffmeyer A, Kroger JC, Freund M, Hain J, Holle A *et al.* Microencapsulated cell-mediated treatment of inoperable pancreatic carcinoma. Lancet 2001; 357: 1591-2.

[94]   Sakai S, Kawabata K, Tanaka S, Harimoto N, Hashimoto I, Mu C *et al.* Subsieve-size agarose capsules enclosing ifosfamide-activating cells: a strategy toward chemotherapeutic targeting to tumors. Mol Cancer Ther 2005; 4: 1786-90.

[95]   Sakai S, Hashimoto I, Tanaka S, Salmons B, Kawakami K. Small agarose microcapsules with cell-enclosing hollow core for cell therapy: Transplantation of ifosfamide-activating cells to the mice with pre-established subcutaneous tumor. Cell Transplant. 2009; 18:933-9.

INDEX

A

Adenosine triphosphate 15, 18

Advanced therapy 70, 81

Agarose 11, 32, 71, 109, 144, 153, 158-161

Aggregates 3, 106

Aggregation 14, 34

Alginate 22, 30, 55, 62, 70, 87, 102, 134, 162, 163

Alginate lyase 153, 165, 167

Alginate with phenolic moieties 153

Allogeneic stem cell 79, 86

Alternating magnetic field 93, 97

Alzheimer's disease 102, 147, 148

Amyotrophic lateral sclerosis 102, 109, 110, 113, 123, 125, 141, 143, 148

Antibodies 10, 23, 53, 58, 70, 72, 77, 107, 132

Anti-idiotypic response 74

Apoptosis 9, 15, 25, 82, 85, 118, 123, 134

Arginine challenge test 49, 50, 52

Autoimmunity 8, 59

B

Barium alginate 40, 43, 59, 64, 66

B-cell activation by encapsulated cells 73

Beta cell 41, 49, 55, 60

Bioartificial pancreas 26, 31, 37, 67-69, 172, 175

Biocompatibility 19, 22, 29, 70, 71, 106, 153, 154, 160

Bioencapsulation 70, 107

Biomaterial 22, 29, 102, 108-109, 138, 140, 154

Biomolecule release 70

Blood 3, 20, 25, 44, 60, 79, 86, 127, 134

Blood brain barrier 104

Blood vessels 9, 20, 23, 57, 82, 134

Brain 86, 102-104, 113, 119, 128, 134, 140

www.ingramcontent.com/pod-product-compliance
Lightning Source LLC
Chambersburg PA
CBHW041702210326
41598CB00007B/501

www.ingramcontent.com/pod-product-compliance
Lightning Source LLC
Chambersburg PA
CBHW070732220326
41598CB00024BA/3401